Comprehensive Virology 1

Comprehensive Virology

Edited by Heinz Fraenkel-Conrat
University of California at Berkeley

and Robert R. Wagner
University of Virginia

Editorial Board

Comprehensive

Edited by

Heinz Fraenkel-Conrat

Department of Molecular Biology and Virus Laboratory
University of California, Berkeley, California

and

Robert R. Wagner

Department of Microbiology
University of Virginia, Charlottesville, Virginia

Virology

1
Descriptive Catalogue of Viruses

PLENUM PRESS • NEW YORK AND LONDON

Library of Congress Cataloging in Publication Data

Fraenkel-Conrat, Heinz, 1910-
  Comprehensive virology.

  Includes bibliographies.
  CONTENTS: v. 1. Descriptive catalogue of viruses.
  1. Virology—Collected works. I. Wagner, Robert R., 1923-   joint
author. II. Title. [DNLM: 1. Virus diseases. 2. Viruses. QW160 F799ca]
QR357.F72   576'.64'08   74-5494
ISBN 0-306-35141-2 (v. 1)

Library of Congress Cataloging in Publication Data

Fraenkel-Conrat, Heinz, 1910-
  Descriptive catalogue of viruses.

  (His Comprehensive virology, v. 1)
  Includes bibliographies.
  1. Viruses — Dictionaries. I. Title. [DNLM: 1. Virus diseases. 2. Viruses.
QW160 F799ca]
QR357.F72 vol. 1 [QR358]   576'.64'08s [576'.64'03]
ISBN 0-306-35141-2   74-5493

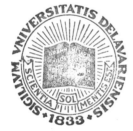

© 1974 Plenum Press, New York
A Division of Plenum Publishing Corporation
227 West 17th Street, New York, N.Y. 10011

United Kingdom edition published by Plenum Press, London
A Division of Plenum Publishing Company, Ltd.
4a Lower John Street, London W1R 3PD, England

Printed in the United States of America

Foreword

The time seems ripe for a critical compendium of that segment of the biological universe we call viruses. Virology, as a science, having only recently passed through its descriptive phase of naming and numbering, has probably reached that stage at which relatively few new—truly new—viruses will be discovered. Triggered by the intellectual probes and techniques of molecular biology, genetics, biochemical cytology, and high-resolution microscopy and spectroscopy, the field has experienced a genuine information explosion.

Few serious attempts have so far been made to chronicle these events. This comprehensive series, which will comprise some 6000 pages in a total of about 22 volumes, represents a commitment by a large group of active investigators to analyze, digest, and expostulate on the great mass of data relating to viruses, much of which is now amorphous and disjointed and scattered throughout a wide literature. In this way, we hope to place the entire field in perspective as well as to develop an invaluable reference and sourcebook for researchers and students at all levels. This series is designed as a continuum that can be entered anywhere but which also provides a logical progression of developing facts and integrated concepts.

The first volume contains an alphabetical catalogue of almost all viruses of vertebrates, insects, plants, and protists, describing them in general terms. Volumes 2–5 will deal primarily, though not exclusively, with the processes of infection and reproduction of the major groups of viruses in their hosts. Volume 2 deals with the simple RNA viruses of bacteria, plants, and animals; the togaviruses (formerly called arboviruses), which share with these only the feature that the virion's RNA is able to act as messenger RNA in the host cell; and the reoviruses of animals and plants, which all share several structurally singular features, the most important being the double-strandedness of their multiple RNA molecules. This grouping, of course, has only slightly more in its favor than others that could have been or indeed were considered.

Volume 3 addresses itself to the reproduction of all DNA-containing viruses of vertebrates, a seemingly simple act of classification, even though the field encompasses the smallest and the largest viruses known.

The reproduction of the larger and more complex RNA viruses represents the subject matter of Volume 4. These share the property of lipid-rich envelopes with the togaviruses included in Volume 2. They share as a group, and with the reoviruses, the presence of enzymes in their virions and the need for their RNA to become transcribed before it can serve messenger functions.

Volume 5 attends to the reproduction of DNA viruses in bacteria, again ranging from small and simple to large and complex.

Aspects of virion structure and assembly of many of these viruses will be dealt with in the following series of volumes, while their genetics, the regulation of their development, viroids, and coviruses will be discussed in subsequently published series. The last volumes will concentrate on host–virus interactions, and on the effects of chemicals and radiation on viruses and their components. At this juncture in the planning of *Comprehensive Virology*, we cannot foresee whether certain topics will become important aspects of the field by the time the final volumes go to press. We envisage the possibility of including volumes on such topics if the need arises.

It is hoped to keep the series at all times up to date by prompt and rapid publication of all contributions, and by encouraging the authors to update their chapters by additions or corrections whenever a volume is reprinted.

Contents

Descriptive Catalogue of Viruses

Heinz Fraenkel-Conrat

*Department of Molecular Biology
and Virus Laboratory
University of California
Berkeley, California*

Introduction

This first volume of *Comprehensive Virology* might be regarded as the list of characters preceding a play, although this list is here to be embellished with a general description of each member of this cast of viruses. It will be attempted to list most of the basic facts, particularly those expressible in numbers, known about all the viruses that have been studied in structural terms. This is a rather formidable undertaking, and it cannot fail to show errors and omissions. But having frequently searched in vain for a concise summary of what is known about a given virus, I believe that this effort is worthwhile for its own sake, quite apart from setting the stage for the subsequent volumes of *Comprehensive Virology*, which will deal in depth with the various properties of viruses.

To make this listing useful requires an organization which enables the searcher to find a given virus without knowing to what class it belongs or to which other viruses it is related. Thus, viruses will be grouped only in terms of viruses of vertebrates and insects, plant viruses, and protist (mostly bacterial) viruses. All will be listed alphabetically, by their complete name(s) or symbol identification.

Virus group names will also be included in the alphabetical list, with a brief description of the characteristics of the group, and reference to typical members of that group. Representative electron micrographs of most virus groups will be shown.*

Most viruses occur as families of more or less closely related strains or serotypes. In most instances only one or a few particularly characteristic representatives of any such family of strains will be separately listed or described.

---

* The author is indebted to Dr. Robley C. Williams for most of the electron micrographs. These were photographed by the minimal beam exposure technique, which is able to disclose finer detail of structure than was heretofore obtained. An atlas showing the best attainable pictures of many viruses is in press (Robley C. Williams and H. W. Fisher, published by Charles C. Thomas). The micrographs incorporated in this catalogue to illustrate the general shapes of various viruses are not intended to show as much fine structure and are at smaller magnification. The micrographs of the corona and arenaviruses were kindly supplied by Dr. F. A. Murphy, that of the alfalfa mosaic virus by Dr. E. M. J. Jaspars and Mrs. M. K. J. Hannaart-Toen.

Only those viruses will be included for which some information concerning physical properties is available (size, shape, chemical nature of the infective principle). Each listing will give to the extent available 1) the name(s) of the virus; 2) its grouping, classification, and relatedness to others; 3) its particle size, shape, and properties; 4) the nature of its nucleic acid; 5) the nature of its protein(s); and 6) some of its biological properties, such as host range, nature of symptoms and disease, virus yield, stability of the infective agent, etc.

In general each entry is intended to be complete; only in the case of amino acid analyses and of amino acid or nucleotide sequences will the reader be referred to summarizing tables or figures.

Most of the parameters and features of each virus were determined repeatedly at different times and with different methods, and rarely are these data in complete agreement. It would be impossible to list, discuss, and evaluate all these data without enlarging the catalogue enormously. I will therefore include only what I regard as the best value, usually the one most recently obtained. Occasionally averaging may seem justified. When there are gross unresolved disagreements, more than one claimed parameter or conclusion will be listed.

Quantitative data from different laboratories or data from the same laboratory published at different times, such as molecular weights of coat proteins, particle weights, etc., frequently agree quite poorly. Thus, while the authors may characterize their set of data by an error of $\pm 2\%$, comparison of different sets of data shows divergences of as much as 20%. Again, I will use my best judgment in giving only one figure, but request the reader to regard all figures as no more than approximations. The number of hard quantitative and agreed-upon facts in the field of virology is quite small, possibly not going much beyond the molecular weights and amino acid and nucleotide sequences of the coat proteins and nucleic acids of TMV and the RNA phages.

To document the sources of the information from which I have drawn would require a very long list of references and at least double the length of this book.The alternative of not listing any references was seriously considered. Finally it was decided to give one or two *recent* references for the more actively studied viruses to facilitate the reader's search for the key data in earlier publications. The references listed are in most instances not the most important sources of data for the given virus. They are not intended to give credit, but only to provide clues.

Viruses of Vertebrates and Insects*

Acado virus (orbivirus subgroup of reoviridiae).

Acute bee-paralysis virus, *see* bee acute paralysis virus.

Acute laryngotracheobronchitis virus (parainfluenza·type 2 virus).

ADENOVIRUSES (a uniform group or genus). Medium large nonenveloped particles of polygonal symmetry, 70–80 nm in diameter, of a density of 1.34 g/ml in CsCl and a particle weight of about 175×10^6 daltons, containing linear double-stranded DNA of $20–23 \times 10^6$ dalton molecular weight. The icosahedral protein shell consists of 240 hexons (each bound to 6 neighbors), and at the apices 12 pentons (each bound to 5 neighbors) which carry fibers. The pentons and hexons are round, 8 nm in diameter, the fiber 20×2 nm with a terminal knob 4 nm in diameter (see Electron micrograph I).

The virus is replicated and assembled in the nucleus. Many adenoviruses are oncogenic, particularly for newborn hamsters and rats, and transform cells in culture. There are 31 known serotypes pathogenic for man (of which types 12, 18, and 31 are highly oncogenic and types 3, 7, 8, 11, 14, 16, and 21 less so in hamsters). There are also many simian adenoviruses, of which SV1, 11, 20, 23, 25, 30, 33, 34, 37, 38, and SA7 are oncogenic, as is an avian serotype (celo) and a bovine serotype (type 3). Canine, porcine, and murine adenoviruses also exist. All mammalian strains share

---

* Many names of animal viruses start, like those of plant viruses, with the host's name (bovine, feline, avian, human, etc.), and frequently this adjective is omitted. The reader is advised to search under both names, with and without this prefix adjective. Also, some general features of virus groups are listed under the group name and not reiterated for each member of the group. Thus the reader is advised to look in both places.

one antigen. Except for the highly oncogenic strains, adenoviruses are very species-specific.

Infection in man may affect the respiratory system, the eyes, or the intestinal tract, often after a period of latency and rarely with serious consequences. Most adenoviruses cause hemagglutination of the erythrocytes of the host or species related to the host.

The nontumorigenic human strains of adenoviruses that have been studied chemically in detail appear very similar or almost identical by the methods used, but the difference between these and the highly oncogenic ones (types 12, 18, 31, which cause tumors in hamsters) is marked in several respects. These two groups will therefore be treated separately in describing structural detail. (Prage and Pettersson, 1971; Prage *et al.*, 1972.)

Human nontumorigenic serotypes (types 2, 4–6, 9, 10, 13, 15, 17, 19, 20, 22–30).

The virus particles (790 S) consist of 87% protein and 13% DNA; their density in CsCl is 1.34 g/ml. The DNA has a molecular weight of 23×10^6 and contains 56–60% (G+C). Its length is about 12 μm. Type 1 adenovirus DNA was found to be slightly infectious for DEAE-treated human embryonic kidney cells.

The main protein, the hexon, amounting to half the weight of the virus, represents trimers of a protein of a molecular weight of 120,000; the other two proteins of the icosahedral shell, penton and fiber, are of dissociated molecular weight 70,000 and 62,000 respectively. The fiber of serotype 2 is 20 nm long with a 4 nm diameter knob. Its undenatured molecular weight is about 200,000.

The dense internal core of the virus (40 nm diameter) contains associated with the DNA about 1000 molecules of a protein rich in arginine (23%) and alanine (20%) of molecular weight 22,000, and less of another of molecular weight 45,000. Three other minor protein components of about 10,000 mol. wt. as well as the 22,000 mol. wt. protein may be host cell histones. For amino acid compositions, see Table 1.

Human tumorigenic serotypes (type 7A, 12, 18, 31).

Differences between the tumorigenic and the nontumorigenic adenoviruses were detected mainly in the DNA, in that the DNA of the tumorigenic strains has a molecular weight of only 21×10^6 and contains 47–49% (G+C); the weakly oncogenic strains (types 2, 3, 7, 8, 11, 14, 16, 21) contain 50–53% (G+C). The lower values of the more oncogenic strains are closer to those of host DNA.

Regarding the proteins, the tumorigenic strains differ from type 2 only in minor detail, suggestive of a few amino acid exchanges in most of the proteins of the virus. (Burlingham and Doerfler, 1972.)

Adeno-associated viruses (AAV) (defective parvoviruses). At least 4 serotypes are known.

Particles of 20–25 nm diameter; 7.5×10^6 particle weight; density in CsCl 1.38–1.44 g/ml. They contain single-stranded DNA of molecular weight 1.6×10^6, either of the two complementary strands being encapsidated in the virion (type 2: A/G/T/C = 21/27/27/26 for one DNA strand and 25/27/22/27 for the other). The main protein, comprising 80%, has a molecular weight of 64,000; two others (10% each) are 77,000 and 90,000.

Adeno-associated viruses replicate in the nucleus only in the presence of certain adenoviruses (and possibly herpesviruses) but are unrelated to these helpers serologically and chemically. The virus is resistant to lipid solvents and many chemicals, as well as to heating (1 hour at 60°C). Types 1–3 do not hemagglutinate; type 4 does hemagglutinate human O erythrocytes at 4°C, but not at 37°C. (Berns and Adler, 1972).

Aedes iridescent virus of mosquitoes, *see* mosquito iridescent viruses.

Aerocystis agent, *see* swim bladder inflammation agent of carp.

African horse sickness virus (orbivirus subgroup of reoviridiae). 60–80 nm diameter. Vector: *Culicoides* spp.

African swinefever virus (icosahedral cytoplasmic DNA virus or possibly iridovirus). Icosahedral particles of about 200 nm diameter but in contrast to iridoviruses covered with an ether-sensitive membrane. The virus contains a dense 80 nm nucleoid. Lethal in domestic pigs, symptomless in the natural host, wild warthogs. (Almeida *et al.,* 1967; Hess, 1971.)

Alastrim (vaccinia virus, subgroup of poxviruses). Very similar, if not identical, to variola minor virus.

Allerton virus, *see* bovine ulcerative mammilitis virus.

ALPHAVIRUS GROUP. Preferred name for group A arboviruses, members of the togaviridiae. Spherical enveloped 40–70 nm diameter particles (240–280 S) containing about 5% single-stranded RNA of $3.4–4.5 \times 10^6$ daltons. Glycoproteins of $63–51 \times 10^3$ and capsid proteins of about 30×10^3 daltons have been reported. Prototype: Sindbis virus. Other members: Aura, Chikungunya, eastern equine encephalitis, Getah, Mayaro, Middleburg, Mucambo,

Ndumu, O'Nyong-nyong, Pixuna, Ross River, Semliki Forest, Una, Venezuelan equine encephalitis, western equine encephalitis, and Whataroa viruses. (Horzinek, 1973.)

Amapari virus (arenavirus).

Amphibian cytoplasmic virus (possible member of iridovirus group).

Amsacta poxvirus (insect poxvirus). Contains 1.5% DNA.

Apoi virus (flavivirus subgroup of togaviridiae).

ARBO(R)VIRUSES. A classifying term which is no longer recommended, covering togaviridiae and many other but not all *arthro*-pod-*bor*ne viruses.

ARENAVIRUS GROUP (or arenoviruses). Poorly defined group of serologically related enveloped RNA viruses 90–220 nm in diameter, with densely spaced surface projections, and dense internal 20–25 nm granules believed to be host ribosomes (see Electron micrograph II). Members: Lassa, lymphocytic choriomeningitis, Machupo, Tacaribe, Junin, Amapari, Pichinde, Parana, Tamiani, Latino, Pistillo viruses. Most arenaviruses cause chronic infections in rodents; some, e.g., Lassa virus, cause acute disease, often fatal, in man and other animals. (Rowe *et al.*, 1970.)

Argentina virus (a strain of vesicular stomatitis virus closely related to Cocal virus).

A-type particles. Particles with toroidal nucleoid resembling oncornaviruses and associated with tumors but not proven to be viral in nature. (Yang and Wivel, 1973.)

Aura virus (alphavirus subgroup of togaviridiae). Related to western equine encephalitis virus. About 50 nm in diameter. Pathogenic for newborn mice.

Australian antigen, *see* hepatitis viruses. (Sukeno *et al.*, 1972)

Avian encephalomyelitis virus (picornavirus of chickens).

Avian herpesviruses (of pigeons, owls, parrots, cormorants); proposed name: phasianid herpesviruses.

Avian infectious bronchitis virus, *see* infectious bronchitis virus.

Avian influenza A virus (myxovirus). Serological differences noted in 10 strains (4 major groups) in regard to neuraminidases and hemagglutinin (*see* influenza viruses). (Madeley *et al.*, 1971.)

AVIAN LEUKOSIS VIRUSES (group of leukoviruses).* Similar in most
respects to murine leukoviruses. Six subgroups have been identified.
The properties of all these viruses are exemplified by the prototype,
avian myeloblastosis virus (see below). They are transformation-defective and contain slightly smaller RNA molecules than nondefective strains causing tumors and focus formation (transformation)
of fibroblasts (*see* Rous sarcoma virus).

Avian myeloblastosis virus (AMV) (prototype avian leukosis virus).
Pleomorphic particles 80 nm in diameter (about 500×10^6 dalton
particle weight), consisting of a dense 40 nm possibly icosahedral
capsid, and a membrane or envelope studded with spikes or knobs.
The envelope is largely derived from the host cell plasma
membrane and is rich in the enzymes occurring in that membrane
(e.g., ATPase). The virus capsid is assembled in the cytoplasm, but
the RNA is probably replicated in the nucleus with an intermediate
stage of DNA synthesis. Thus the virus, like all oncornaviruses,
contains RNA-dependent DNA polymerase (reverse transcriptase).*
The virus matures as it buds through the plasma membrane. Its lipids but not its envelope proteins are probably derived from that
membrane. The virus is sensitive to ether.

The capsid contains single-stranded RNA, $10-12 \times 10^6$ daltons
per particle, 60–65 S, as well as smaller RNAs (10–12 S, 5 S, 4 S).
Upon heating or other means of separating paired bases, the large
RNA is dissociated to 30–35 S, as well as smaller material (12 S–
4 S). Thus the genome is believed to exist in 3 or 4 pieces of $2.5-4 \times
10^6$ mol. wt., held together by short H-bonded segments. The
average composition is $A/G/U/C = 25/29/23/23$. The 3′-termini
of the 30–35 S RNA are predominantly unphosphorylated adenosine with lesser amounts of cytidine and uridine. The 4 S RNA is
probably in part tRNA.

The main proteins of the envelope are two glycoproteins (37,000
and 115,000 mol. wt.), the type-specific antigens. The purified core
largely consists of a protein of 24,000–28,000 mol. wt. This and a
protein of 12,000 mol. wt. represent the group-specific antigens.

The lipids of the envelope are qualitatively the same and quantitatively similar to those of the host cell's plasma membrane. The
core retains most of the DNA-polymerase and reverse transciptase
activities characteristically occurring in all oncornaviruses. The
core also is slightly infectious; it contains the RNA in the 62 S

* See footnote on page 34.

form but also some (< 5%) 27 S and 17 S cellular RNA and 4–5 S RNA.

Avian leukosis viruses cause widespread infection in domestic chickens, at times leading to visceral lymphomatosis, but often remaining symptomless. (Stromberg, 1972; Bolognesi *et al.*, 1972.)

Avian reticuloendotheliosis virus, *see* reticuloendotheliosis virus.

Avian sarcoma viruses, *see* Rous sarcoma virus.

B virus of monkeys (proposed name: cercopithecid herpesvirus).

B 77 (nondefective avian Rous sarcoma virus strain).

B 1327 virus (orbivirus subgroup of reoviridiae).

Baculovirus group. Proposed name for nuclear polyhedrosis and granulosis viruses; *see* under these names.

Bahig, Bakan, Banzi, Batai viruses (either flaviviruses or Bunyamwera supergroup, both subgroups of togaviridiae).

Bat salivary virus, *see* salivary virus.

BeAr 35646, BeAr 41067 (orbivirus subgroup of reoviridiae).

Bebaru virus (alphavirus subgroup of togaviridiae).

Bee acute paralysis virus (nonoccluded insect picornavirus). 28 nm diameter particles (160 S) of buoyant density in CsCl 1.34 g/ml. Contains 25% single-stranded RNA (30 S), 2×10^6 mol. wt. A/G/U/C = 30/19/30/21. Infects only the adult insects. (Newman *et al.*, 1973.)

Bee chronic paralysis virus (unclassified insect virus). Ellipsoid particles 22×41, 54, and 64 nm (97 S, 110 S, 125 S), not ether sensitive, containing RNA.

Bhanga virus (either flavivirus or Bunyamwera supergroup, both subgroups of togaviridiae).

Birdpox viruses (subgroup of poxviruses, including fowlpox, canarypox, pigeonpox, turkeypox, etc.). Double-stranded DNA of 200×10^6 mol. wt.

Bittner virus, *see* mouse mammary tumor virus.

Bluetongue virus of sheep (orbivirus subgroup of reoviridiae). Two types, 69 and 63 nm particles (550 S and 490 S), probably composed of a single shell of 32 capsomeres with a 23 nm central nucleoid (density 1.36 and 1.38 g/ml in CsCl). The virus contains

20% of double-stranded RNA, probably 10 components, 42% (G+C) on average. The largest component has a molecular weight of 2.7×10^6, the total RNA of the particle being about 12×10^6 daltons. Four major and three minor capsid proteins (110, 100, 58, 32×10^3; and 155, 72, and 38×10^3) corresponding in molecular weight to respective RNA components. The smaller particles lack the 110 and 58×10^3 surface components. They are less infective but contain transcriptase, which is not detectable in the larger component. Transmitted by *Culicoides* spp. The virus replicates also in vector, causes severe disease in sheep. (Martin and Zweerink, 1972; Verwoerd *et al.*, 1972.) (The differences between orbiviruses and classical reoviruses are diminishing as more is being learned about them.)

Bovine adenovirus, *see* adenovirus.

Bovine diarrhea virus (unclassified, possibly flavivirus subgroup of togaviridiae). 57 nm particles with 25 nm core. Sensitive to ether; density in CsCl 1.15 g/ml. Contains RNA.

Bovine enterovirus VG-5-27 (enterovirus subgroup of picornaviridiae). 28 nm diameter particle (165 S); density in CsCl 1.34 g/ml; contains single-stranded RNA of 2.8×10^6 mol. wt. (35 S). Four equimolar proteins: 34,000, 28,000, 26,000, and 7300 mol. wt. The 75 S procapsid lacks the smallest protein component (*see* mouse-Elberfeld virus for viral architecture). (Martin and Johnston, 1972.)

Bovine ephemeral (or epizootic) fever virus (not yet classified). Bullet-shaped (140×80 nm) and conical (176×88 nm) particles. The virus has a density of 1.19 g/ml in CsCl; it is ether sensitive but it contains a 12 S double-stranded RNA. (Tanaka *et al.*, 1969, 1972.)

Bovine lumpy skin disease virus (paravaccinia virus subgroup of poxviruses).

Bovine mammilitis virus (bovid herpesvirus 2). 64% (G+C).

Bovine papilloma virus, *see* papilloma virus.

Bovine papular stomatitis virus (paravaccinia subgroup of poxviruses, related to orf virus).

Bovine parainfluenza virus (type 3 parainfluenza virus subgroup of paramyxoviruses). Many serotypes. 280–580 nm particles containing an 18 nm helical nucleocapsid. Causes shipping fever.

Bovine respirating syncytial virus (*see also* respiratory syncytial virus). Particles of 110 nm diameter with 15 nm projections, and helical nucleocapsid of about 13 nm diameter (Malmquist *et al.*, 1969; Ito *et al.*, 1973b.)

Bovine rhinotracheitis virus, *see* infectious bovine rhinotracheitis.

Bovine ulcerative mammilitis virus (Allerton virus) (herpesvirus).

B particles, *see* B-type virus.

Brazil virus (strain of vesicular stomatitis virus).

Brazilian myxomavirus (myxoma subgroup of poxviruses).

Bryan strain of Rous sarcoma virus (replication-defective, usually contains RAV) (*see* Rous sarcoma virus).

B-type virus, *see* mouse mammary tumor virus.

Buffalopox virus (vaccinia virus). Closely related to cowpox virus, but distinguishable.

Bukalasa virus (flavivirus subgroup of togaviridiae).

BUNYAMWERA SUPERGROUP VIRUSES (not yet clearly reclassified "arboviruses"). At least 9 serotypes, 60–120 nm diameter. Batai and Inkoo viruses are spherical enveloped particles, 60 and 55 nm in diameter, excluding 12 and 15 nm projections respectively. They contain a helical nucleocapsid, similar to that of Uukuniemi virus. These helices differentiate the Bunyamwera group from typical togaviruses (Semliki Forest and Sindbis viruses), and their appearance is also clearly different from the myxovirus nucleocapsids. (Holmes, 1971.)

Bussuquara, Bwamba viruses (togaviridiae).

Cache Valley virus (member of Bunyamwera supergroup of togaviridiae).

CALICIVIRUS GROUP (subgroup of picornaviridiae). Larger than other subgroups (37 nm diameter, 175 S). Members: Vesicular exanthema and some feline viruses. Buoyant density in CsCl 1.37 g/ml (more than entero- and cardioviruses and less than rhino- and foot and mouth disease viruses). Contain 22% RNA and a 63×10^3 protein.

California encephalitis viruses (human alphaviruses or more probably members of the Bunyamwera viruses, exemplified by LaCross virus). Particles of 95 nm diameter. The 12 nm envelope matures during release of the virus. (Lyons and Heyduk, 1973.)

California myxoma virus (myxoma subgroup of poxviruses).

Canarypox virus (birdpox subgroup of poxviruses).

Candivu virus (togavirus).

Canine distemper virus (paramyxovirus). Closely related to measles and rinderpest virus. Pleomorphic particles of predominantly 200–250 nm diameter, with about 7-nm-thick outer membrane and 11 nm projections. The helical nucleocapsid has a diameter of 15–18 nm and a 5 nm axial canal. Buoyant density in CsCl 1.23 g/ml. The virus lacks neuraminidase. (Appel and Gillespie, 1972.)

Canine hepatitis virus (adenovirus).

Canine herpesvirus 61% (G+C).

Canine papilloma virus 300 S and 165 S for full and empty capsids.

Cardiovirus group (subgroup related to enteroviruses of picornaviridiae). Members: Mengo virus, encephalomyocarditis virus, mouse-Elberfeld virus, etc. Density 1.32–1.34 g/ml, stable over the range of pH 3–10; 151–162 S. (Eggen and Shatkin, 1972.)

Carr–Zilber Rous sarcoma virus (nondefective avian sarcoma virus).

Celo virus, *see* chick embryo lethal orphan virus.

Central European tick-borne encephalitis virus (togavirus).

CH 9935 (orbivirus subgroup of reoviridiae).

Chandiporna virus (human rhabdovirus).

Changuinola virus (orbivirus subgroup of reoviridiae).

Channel catfish virus (herpesvirus). 175–200 nm particles of icosahedral symmetry, 162 capsomeres. The virus becomes enveloped at the nuclear membrane. (Wolf and Darlington, 1972.)

Chenuda virus (orbivirus subgroup of reoviridiae).

Chick embryo lethal orphan virus (celo virus) (oncogenic avian adenovirus). 60–80 nm icosahedral particles, 252 capsomeres. Density in CsCl 1.35 or 1.32 g/ml. DNA, 17.3%, of 30×10^6 mol. wt. It is unique, nonpermuted, linear, and double-stranded, lacks cohesive ends, and contains 54% or 46% (G+C). The virions are 81% protein, similar to other adenoviruses, except that the pentons are quite different from those of human adenovirus and carry two fibers of 43 and 9 nm length. (For amino acid analysis of the hexon, see Table 1). (Laver *et al.,* 1971.)

Chicken herpesvirus 45% (G+C).

Chickenpox virus (human herpesvirus 3) *see* varicella–zoster virus.

Chick syncytial virus (oncornavirus, related to reticuloendotheliosis virus).

Chikungunya virus (alphavirus subgroup of togaviridiae).

Chilo iridescent virus (insect iridovirus).

Citrus red mite virus (picornavirus).

Cocal virus (rhabdovirus of mite). 60 × 170 nm bullet-shaped particles. Genetically and serologically related to vesicular stomatitis virus; Indiana serotype.

Coital exanthema virus, equine herpesvirus 3.

Colorado tick fever virus (orbivirus subgroup of reoviridiae). Not enveloped particles containing double-stranded RNA. Vector: *Dermacentor* spp. Host: man (virus replicates in both).

Columbia SK virus (cardiovirus subgroup of picornaviridiae). Related to encephalomyocarditis, mouse-Elberfeld virus, etc.

Congo virus (togavirus).

Contagious pustular dermatitis virus (paravaccinia subgroup of poxviruses, related to orf virus).

CORONAVIRUS GROUP. Recently defined group of viruses resembling myxoviruses, the most marked distinguishing characteristics being 20-nm-long, widely spaced club-shaped or petal-shaped projections, instead of spikes, which give the particles their corona-like appearance. The entire virus maturation appears to occur in the cytoplasm, not through budding. Human prototype OC 43: 390 S particles, 80–160 nm in diameter, particle weight 112×10^6 daltons. The clublike projections are 15–20 nm long, 10 nm across the wide part (see Electron micrograph III).

The membrane appears to be double. The virus is ether and acid sensitive. Its buoyant density in CsCl is 1.19 g/ml. The 7–8 nm threadlike nucleocapsids (similar to those of myxoviruses) contain single-stranded RNA.

The proteins are a nucleocapsid protein (26%) of 30,000 mol. wt., and an envelope glycoprotein and protein of 104,000 (8%) and 47,000 (16%). Other proteins not yet located but surely mostly from the envelope are a glycolipoprotein of 191,000 mol. wt. (13%) and two glycoproteins of 60,000 and 15,000 (23% and 14%).

Besides many human serotypes (often found in association with common colds), other members of the corona virus group are avian infectious bronchitis virus, murine hepatitis virus, transmissible gastroenteritis and hemagglutinating encephalomyelitis viruses of pigs, pneumotropic virus of rats, etc. In man these viruses usually give respiratory symptoms. (Hierholzer *et al.*, 1972.)

Corriparta virus (insect orbivirus, subgroup of reoviridiae). Host: *Culex mosquito.*

Coryza virus (rhinovirus subgroup of picornaviridiae).

Cowbone ridge virus (flavivirus).

Cowpox virus (subgroup I poxvirus), *see* under poxvirus.

Coxsackie virus (enterovirus subgroup of picornaviridiae). A: 24 serotypes; B: 6 serotypes. Particles of 153 S, 28 nm diameter, and a particle weight of about 7×10^6, containing about 30% single-stranded RNA. A/G/U/C = 28/28/24/20. The particles consist of four proteins, like other enteroviruses. Serotype A7 is neurotropic in man. (Tannock *et al.*, 1970.)

C particles, *see* C-type viruses.

Creutzfeld–Jakob disease agent of man, *see* slow viruses, scrapie.

Cricket virus (picornavirus).

Croup-associated virus, *see* parainfluenza viruses.

Crystalline array virus of grasshoppers (picornavirus). Particles of less than 25 nm diameter.

C-type viruses, term used for all oncornaviruses with centrally located spherical nucleoid, i.e., all except the mouse mammary tumor virus (B-type).

Cytomegaloviruses (*see* human herpesvirus 5 and other herpesviruses). Associated with salivary gland of man, guinea pig, mouse, swine, vervet, horse. DNA of 100×10^6 daltons (55 S); composition of the human virus: 57% (G+C); vervet virus, 51% (G+C); mouse virus, 59% (G+C), 132×10^6 molecular weight. (Huang *et al.*, 1973.)

Cytoplasmic polyhedrosis viruses (occluded isometric diplornaviruses of insects, e.g., silkworm). Polyhedral inclusion bodies 0.5–15 μm in diameter consisting predominantly of 2 proteins of 30,000 and 20,000 mol. wt. Embedded in this matrix are many icosahedral virus particles 60–65 nm in diameter, with large knobs, not enveloped. The virus is of about 400 S and 2.9×10^7 particle weight; its buoyant density in CsCl is 1.435 g/ml. The RNA of the *Bombyx mori* virus (12.7×10^6 daltons total) occurs in 10 double strands, all $3'$ terminating in U and C followed by a pyrimidine. Their molecular weights range from 2.7 to 0.37×10^6 daltons; average composition: $A/G/U/C = 28/22/29/21$. The RNA of the *Malacosoma distria* virus totals 20.3×10^6 daltons.

The virion proteins have molecular weights of 151, 142, 130, 67, and 33×10^3, but the proteins of the polyhedron matrix may also be virus coded (molecular weight 122, 100, 48, 30, and 20×10^3).

The virions contain RNA polymerase which is able quickly to transcribe each of the RNA components. The virus hemagglutinates mammalian cells. (Lewandowski and Traynor, 1972; Shimotohno and Miura, 1973.)

D'Anguilar virus (orbivirus subgroup of reoviridiae).

Dakar bat virus (flavivirus).

Deer fibroma virus (papilloma virus).

Defective viruses. Many different RNA and DNA viruses have been found to occur in lighter and noninfective forms, usually due to a deficiency of nucleic acid. Such phenomena have particularly been studied with influenza virus (von Magnus particles), Sendai virus, vesicular stomatitis virus, reovirus, adenovirus, and herpesvirus. Virions lacking nucleic acid ("top components") have also been observed, as well as virions containing host DNA instead of viral DNA (pseudoviruses). (Huang *et al.*, 1966; von Magnus, 1954; Schlesinger, 1969; Kingsbury *et al.*, 1970; Mak, 1971; Nonoyama *et al.*, 1970.)

Dengue virus (flavivirus subgroup of togaviridiae). Four known serotypes: Dengue virus 2: spherical 50 nm particles with 26 nm core. Single-stranded RNA (45 S), $A/G/U/C = 31/26/22/21$. Nucleocapsid protein of 13,500 mol. wt. (lysine rich, histidine deficient); the envelope glycoproteins of 59,000 mol. wt.; and a membranous capsid protein tightly bound to the envelope of 8000 mol. wt. (Stollar, 1969; Matsumura *et al.*, 1971.)

Densonucleosis virus (*Galleria* dense nuclear virus) (insect parvovirus). Particles of 22 nm diameter consisting of 42 capsomeres; density in CsCl 1.440 g/ml; contains 37% DNA, probably single-stranded within the virion, of 2×10^6 mol. wt. and buoyant density of 1.711 g/ml in CsCl. (Kurstak *et al.*, 1973.)

DIPLORNAVIRUS GROUP. Not yet officially accepted name for double-stranded RNA viruses (reoviridiae). This is a group of viruses occurring in man, mammals, plants, and insects (the latter not acting as vectors but regular hosts). The plant diplornaviruses (e.g., rice dwarf virus and wound tumor virus) will be dealt with in Section B; they are very similar in most respects to the diplornaviruses infecting animals and insects.

These viruses are characterized by single or more often double shells of protein, therefore of either about 60 or 80 nm diameter, of cubic symmetry, and lacking an envelope and thus not ether sensitive (see Electron micrograph IV). They contain 10–15 molecules of double-stranded RNA (diplo-RNA). The two animal subgroups of diplornaviridiae known are the reoviruses and the orbiviruses (bluetongue virus). The diplornaviruses, like possibly all groups of RNA viruses except the picorna- and togaviridiae, carry their own transcriptase.

Members of the animal and insect diplornavirus group are the reoviruses, African horse sickness, bluetongue, Changuinola, Colorado tick fever, Corriparta, epizootic hemorrhagic disease of deer, epizootic diarrhea of mice, Eubenangee, infectious pancreatic necrosis of trout, Kemerovo, etc., viruses.

Distemper virus of dogs, *see* canine distemper virus.

Drosophila P virus (insect picornavirus).

Drosophila sigma virus (insect rhabdovirus).

Duck hepatitis virus (enterovirus).

Duck infectious anemia virus (oncornavirus). Related to reticuloendotheliosis virus.

Duck plague virus, probably a herpesvirus (anatid herpesvirus 1). (Hess and Dardiri, 1968.)

Duck spleen necrosis virus (oncornavirus). Related to reticuloendotheliosis virus.

Eastern equine encephalitis virus (EEE) (alphavirus subgroup of togaviridiae). 54 nm particles, 240 S, 58×10^6 particle weight; density in CsCl 1.21 g/ml; lipid-containing envelope. Single-stranded RNA, containing, as probably all togaviridiae, poly(A) sequences, probably 3′ terminal. Multiplies in cytoplasm, matures by budding, in vertebrates and arthropods. (Karabatsos, 1973.)

EB virus, *see* Epstein–Barr virus.

Echo viruses (enterovirus subgroup of picornaviridiae) (*enteric, cyto*pathic *h*uman *o*rphan viruses). 30 serotypes. 27 nm diameter particles of 157 S. Produce no distinct disease.

Echo virus 10 (reovirus).

Echo virus 28 (rhinovirus subgroup of picornaviridiae).

Ectromelia virus, mousepox virus (vaccinia subgroup of poxviruses).

Edgehill virus (flavivirus subgroup of togaviridiae).

Egtved virus of rainbow trout (rhabdovirus). 65 × 180 nm bulletshaped particles.

Encephalomyocarditis virus (EMC) (cardiovirus subgroup of picornaviridiae). About 27 nm diameter particles, 160 S, 8.5×10^6 in particle weight. Density in CsCl 1.34 g/ml. Contains 31.7% singlestranded RNA of 2.6×10^6 mol. wt., A/G/U/C = 26/24/25/25. The RNA contains poly(A), about 58 residues long. Four probably equimolar proteins of 35,000, 28,000, 24,000, and 7000 mol. wt. For comparative data on amino acid composition of three main proteins of EMC and ME virus, see Table 1. One liter culture fluid yields 2–3 mg pure virus. Specific infectivity (particle/PFU) = 20 to 250. (Butterworth and Rueckert, 1972.)

Englebreth–Holm Rous sarcoma virus, *see* Rous sarcoma virus.

Entebbe bat salivary gland virus (flavivirus subgroup of togaviridiae).

ENTEROVIRUS GROUP (subgroup of picornaviridiae). Related to cardioviruses; of same physical properties and stability. Icosahedral particles of about 27 nm diameter; 8.6×10^6 daltons particle weight; 155 S; 1.34 g/ml buoyant density in CsCl; containing 29% single-stranded RNA of 2.6×10^6 daltons. Human, bovine, porcine, avian, and murine species are known.

Entomo poxviruses, *see* insect poxviruses.

Epizootic diarrhea virus of infant mice (related to reovirus).

Epizootic hemorrhagic disease virus of deer (orbivirus subgroup of reoviridiae).

Epstein–Barr virus (human herpesvirus 4). Contains 9% doublestranded DNA of 95×10^6 daltons; density in CsCl 1.718 g/ml, 59% (G+C). Virus isolated from established cell lines of Burkitt lymphoblasts, thus virus apparently associated with human malignancy. The virus is the causative agent of infectious mononucleosis. (Moss and Pope, 1972.)

Equine abortion virus, *see* equine herpesvirus 1.

Equine arteritis virus (probably alphavirus subgroup of togaviridiae, similar to rubella virus). Enveloped, ether sensitive, 57 nm particles, buoyant density in CsCl of 1.18 g/ml. The 25 nm core contains RNA; there are 9 structural proteins (72,000 to 10,500), the major ones being 15,000 and 13,000 in molecular weight. This is similar to the protein pattern of flaviviruses, whereas rubella resembles alphaviruses more closely. (Hyllseth, 1973.)

Equine encephalitis virus, *see* eastern and western equine encephalitis viruses.

Equine herpesvirus 1 (equine abortion or rhinopneumonitis virus). Density of the DNA 1.717 g/ml, 92×10^6 mol. wt.; 58% (G+C). The virus contains about 20 proteins (13,000–115,000 mol. wt.), the nucleocapsid 3; three envelope proteins contain lipid, and four are glycoproteins.

Equine herpesvirus 2 (cytomegalovirus, possibly identical to equine infectious anemia virus). Density of DNA 1.716–1.717 g/ml; 57–58% (G+C).

Equine herpesvirus 3, coital exanthema virus.

Equine infectious anemia virus (possibly belonging to the slow virus group) (from horse leukocytes). Pleomorphic particles of 90–140 nm diameter, with a 40–60 nm core and a 9 nm envelope. Density 1.15 g/ml in CsCl. Ether sensitive. The virus contains RNA. (Nakajima *et al.,* 1970.)

Equine infectious arteritis virus, *see* equine arteritis virus.

Equine rhinopneumonitis virus, *see* equine abortion virus.

Eubenangee virus (orbivirus subgroup of reoviridiae).

FAV-1, *see* frog adenovirus.

Feline ataxia virus (parvovirus).

Feline herpesvirus (probably identical with feline rhinotracheitis virus). 47% (G+C).

Feline leukemia-sarcoma viruses (oncornaviruses). 100 nm particles, containing 75 S single-stranded RNA which upon melting becomes 37 S. A/G/U/C = 30/25/22/23. The 4 S RNA also associated with the virus shows A/G/U/C = 18/33/21/29. The major proteins (15,000, 18,000, and 33,000 mol. wt.) resemble those of murine leukoviruses more than those of avian myeloblastosis virus.

Feline panleucopenia virus (parvovirus).

Feline picornavirus. Density 1.38 g/ml.

Feline rhinotracheitis virus (feline herpesvirus 1). 46% (G+C).

Fibroma virus of rabbits, squirrels, hares (myxoma subgroup of poxviruses).

Fishpox virus (vaccinia subgroup of poxviruses).

Flanders (Hart Park) virus (rhabdovirus of birds and arthropods, not serologically related to others). 218 × 65 nm bullet-shaped particles.

FLAVIVIRUS (OR FLAVO) GROUP. Preferred name for group B arboviruses, subgroup of the togaviridiae. Spherical enveloped particles of 30–55 nm diameter (200 S) containing 7–8% single-stranded RNA of $3-4 \times 10^6$ daltons. Glycoproteins of $65-51 \times 10^3$ and capsid proteins of about 16 and 9×10^3 daltons. (Horzinek, 1973.) Prototype: Yellow fever virus; others: Apoi, Banzi, Bukalasa bat, Bussuquara, Cowbone Ridge, Dakar bat, Dengue, Edgehill, Entebbe bat salivary gland, Ilhéus, Israel turkey meningoencephalitis, Japanese encephalitis, Kokobera, Kunjin, Kyasanur Forest, Langat, louping ill, Modoc, Montana myotis leukoencephalitis, Murray Valley encephalitis, Negishi, Ntaya, Omsk hemorrhagic fever (types I and II), Powassan, Spondweni, St. Louis encephalitis, Stratford, tick-borne encephalitis (subtypes central European and Far Eastern), Uganda S, salivary virus of bats (US), Usutu, Wesselsbron, West Nile, and Zika viruses.

Foamy virus of monkeys and chimpanzees (possibly related to slow viruses, oncornaviruses, or—less likely—togaviruses). At least 7 serotypes known. Type 1 and 2 (strain MK5) contain 35 nm nucleoid and 2 shells, 60 and 90 nm in diameter.

Foot and mouth disease virus (picornavirus). Rhinovirus subgroup of 7 known serotypes. Particles of 27–30 nm diameter of probably the same architecture as mouse-Elberfeld virus (ME); particle weight 8.5×10^6 (140 S). Buoyant density in CsCl 1.43 g/ml (with decomposition to 1.51 g/ml). Virus contains 30–32% single-stranded

RNA, of about 2.5×10^6 dalton molecular weight; $A/G/U/C =$ 26/24/22/28. Four proteins build up the virion, probably in equimolar amounts (60 molecules of each per particle), about 34,000, 29,000, 26,000, and 7000 mol. wt., probably adding up to 96,000. Three different N-terminal amino acids (leucine, isoleucine, and threonine) were found in the virus. The C-terminals were for the three largest proteins, -Glu-Ala-Leu, -Leu-Glu, and -Ser-Glu. For amino acid analyses, see Table 1. The virus degrades at very low ionic strength and below pH 7. (vande Woude and Bachrach, 1971; Bachrach *et al.*, 1973.)

Fowlplague virus (influenza A subgroup of myxoviruses). Three glycoproteins in spikes; glycolipid and three proteins remain after removal of spikes. The hemagglutinin glycoproteins which arise through posttranslational cleavage are 49,000 and 32,000 in molecular weight (18 and 11%), the neuraminidase (7%) 45,000, and the nonglycoproteins (making up 34, 22, and 2%) 26,5000, 60,000, and 84,000. The first two of these represent the membrane and capsid proteins (*see* influenza virus). (Madeley *et al.*, 1971; Klenk and Rott, 1973.)

Fowlpox virus (birdpox subgroup of poxviruses). Contains 28 proteins, most of them identical in molecular weight to those of vaccinia virus.

Friend murine leukemia virus, *see* murine leukemia virus.

Frog adenovirus 1 (not serologically related to other adenoviruses, not oncogenic). (Clark *et al.*, 1973.)

Frog viruses 2 and 3 (FV2, 3) (polyhedral cytoplasmic DNA viruses, probably iridoviruses). Replicate in amphibian and mammalian cells below 37°C. Density of FV3 in CsCl about 1.27 g/ml. The virus consists of 56% protein, 14% lipid, and 30% DNA. The DNA is 57% (G+C), and about 130×10^6 in molecular weight.

In FV3 16 proteins were detected, the main components of which have molecular weights of 49,000, 13,000, 10,500, and 8500 (all 1300–2000 molecules per particle). Various enzyme activities are also found associated with the virion (e.g., ATPase) or with the core nucleocapsid (endonuclease). (Tan and McAuslan, 1971; Aubertin *et al.*, 1971.)

Frog virus 4 (ranid herpesvirus 2). This virus is associated with the Lucké adenocarcinoma virus in frog tumors. 55% (G+C). (Granoff, 1972.)

Fujinami sarcoma virus (oncornavirus).

G 8886, G 15534 (orbivirus subgroup of reoviridiae).

Galleria dense nuclear virus, *see* densonucleosis virus.

Gallus adeno-like virus (GAL virus) (chicken adenovirus).

Gecko virus (possibly a member of iridovirus group).

Getah virus (alphavirus).

Gibbon leukosisvirus (oncornavirus).

Goatpox virus (sheeppox subgroup of poxviruses).

Gomphrena virus (rhabdovirus).

Gonometa virus (insect enterovirus subgroup of picornaviridiae). Particles of 32 nm diameter, 180 S, and density in CsCl 1.35 g/ml. Contains 37% RNA and four proteins of molecular weight of 37,000–12,000. Host: *Gonometa podocarpi.* (Longworth *et al.*, 1973.)

Graffi murine leukemia virus, *see* murine leukemia virus.

Granulosis virus of insects (member of baculovirus group), similar to nuclear polyhedrosis viruses, but singly occluded. The granulosis virus of *Trichoplusiani* contains closed double-stranded supercoiled circular DNA (95 S), relaxed circular DNA (74 S), and linear DNA (60 S). The molecular weight is 100×10^6. (Summers and Anderson, 1972.)

Gross virus (transformation-defective strain of murine leukemia virus).

Guineapig herpesvirus (caviid herpesvirus). Icosahedral particle with double-layered membrane, 166 nm in diameter, with dense core of 101 nm diameter. DNA of density 1.716 g/ml (human herpesvirus 1: 1.728, host DNA 1.700). Always found together with C-type particles in leukemic guinea pigs.

H-1, H-2, H-3 viruses (hamster and rat osteolytic virus) (parvovirus). Particles of 19 nm diameter and buoyant density 1.400 g/ml in CsCl. Contain single-stranded DNA of 28 S (denatured 17 S) and density in CsCl of 1.72 g/ml, 1.7×10^6 mol. wt., A/G/T/C = 26/23/29/23 (like all parvoviruses and mammalian DNA, low in CpG sequence).

Haden virus, *see* hemadsorbing enteric virus.

Hamster papilloma virus, *see* papilloma virus.

Hare fibroma virus (myxoma subgroup of poxviruses).

Hart Park virus (rhabdovirus), *see* Flanders Hart Park virus.

Harvey sarcoma virus, *see* murine sarcoma virus.

Hemadsorbing enteric virus (haden) (bovine parvovirus). Particles of 22.5 nm diameter; density 1.425 g/ml (also a component of 1.45 g/ml and one of empty particles of 1.30 g/ml density). The main protein is of 67,000 daltons. (Johnson and Hoggan, 1973).

Hemadsorption virus 1, 2, *see* parainfluenza viruses.

Hemagglutinating encephalomyelitis virus of pigs (coronavirus). Isometric particle, about 150 nm diameter, including club-shaped 15-nm-long projections. (Clarke and McFerran, 1971.)

Hemagglutinating virus of Japan, *see* Sendai virus.

Hemorrhagic encephalopathy virus (HER) (parvovirus).

Hemorrhagic fever virus (arenavirus). Particles of 60–280 nm diameter with 20–25 nm electron-dense granules (possibly host ribosomes).

Hemorrhagic septicemia agent of salmon (rhabdovirus). (Bachmann and Ahne, 1973.)

Hepatitis viruses A and B (infective and serum hepatitis agents, respectively). Hepatitis B is associated with virus-like particles which have not yet been definitely shown to contain a nucleic acid. These 42 nm particles contain a 27 nm core which is able to bind antibody molecules from the serum of hepatitis patients. Relationship of hepatitis B virus to Australia antigen (hepatitis-associated antigen), a lipoprotein particle, is not yet clear. Viruslike particles of 27nm diameter were found associated with hepatitis A. Relationship of hepatitis virus A to parvoviruses has also been suggested. (Dreesman *et al.,* 1972a; Feinstone *et al.,* 1973.)

Herpesvirus ateles of monkey. Oncogenic *in vivo* and possibly *in vitro.* (Meléndez *et al.,* 1971.)

Herpesvirus cuniculi (rabbit herpesvirus).

HERPESVIRUS GROUP. Large isometric particles of about 150 nm diameter, usually enveloped and ether sensitive; they contain 7% of double-stranded linear DNA of $80-100 \times 10^6$ daltons, 57–74% (G+C). The icosahedral capsid of 100 nm diameter consists of 162 hollow capsomeres. Many herpesviruses are or tend to become oncogenic (*see* Lucké virus, herpesvirus saimiri, Epstein–Barr virus). While the protein is synthesized in the cytoplasm, synthesis of the DNA and assembly of the virion begins in the nucleus. The virus derives its inner envelope largely from the nuclear plasma membrane, including nonprotein host material. An outer envelope forms at the cytoplasmic membrane. Herpesviruses show great changes in virulence, in both directions, when infecting other than natural hosts. (*See also* under herpes simplex virus.)

Herpesvirus saimiri (cebid herpesvirus 2). Produces malignant lymphomas in adult primates. 69% (G+C).

Herpesvirus simiae, *see* B virus of monkeys.

Herpes simplex virus (prototype of herpesviruses). (Types 1 and 2, to be called human herpesvirus 1, 2; also called facialis and genitalis. There is about 40% homology in the nucleotide sequences of these two groups.) Large, enveloped, spherical particles, 160–200 nm in diameter; particle weight 1400×10^6 daltons. Irregular envelope around icosahedral capsid (100 nm diameter), composed of 162 capsomeres ($T = 16$), 150 hexagonal, 12 pentagonal. Particles without envelopes also occur naturally, as well as particles lacking DNA, leaving a hexagonal toroidal (hollow) core of 74 nm exterior diameter and 18 nm inner diameter and 50 nm high. The capsomeres are hollow prisms (10 nm in diameter, 12.5 nm long, with about 3 nm hole). The DNA content is 7%, the molecular weight probably 81×10^6 (55 S) for both subgroups 1 and 2, although their density in CsCl differs slightly, being 1.726 and 1.728 g/ml, corresponding to 67 and 71% (G+C). The isolated DNA is infective. Of the 33 proteins, ranging from 275×10^3 to 23×10^3 in molecular weight, almost half are glycoproteins. The capsid proteins are of 140×10^3, 110×10^3, 34×10^3, and 20×10^3 daltons, the core protein of 44×10^3 mol. wt. (The amino acid compositions of several of these proteins have been reported.) The protein of molecular weight 110×10^3 is the main capsid protein in rabbits (Meléndez *et al.,* 1972; Dreesman *et al.,* 1972b; Gibson and Roizman, 1972.)

Herpesvirus sylvilagus (cottontail rabbit). Causes benign or malignant lymphoproliferative disease. (Hinze and Chipman, 1972.)

Herpesvirus tamarinus, a cebid (monkey) herpesvirus.

Herpes zoster (human herpesvirus 3), *see* varicella–zoster virus.

Hinze lymphoma virus, a rabbit herpesvirus.

Hogcholera virus, *see* swinefever virus.

Huacho virus (orbivirus subgroup of reoviridiae).

Human adenoviruses, *see* adenovirus.

Human cytomegaloviruses (human herpesvirus 5).

Human papilloma virus (wart virus). The particle (56 nm diameter) consists probably of 72 capsomeres (T = 7) (12 pentamers, 60 hexamers), in skew right-handed configuration. 296 S and 168 S for full and empty capsids. DNA 41% (G+C). (*See also* under papilloma virus).

Human respiratory virus, see coronaviruses.

IbAr 22619 (orbivirus subgroup of reoviridiae).

Ibaraki virus of cattle (orbivirus subgroup of reoviridiae). Icosahedral particles of 55 nm diameter. (Ito *et al.,* 1973a.)

Icosahedral cytoplasmic DNA viruses. Newly defined group including African swinefever virus, frog virus 3, lymphocystis virus, etc. The name describes the common features of these viruses (Kelly and Robertson, 1973.)

Ilhéus virus (flavivirus subgroup of togaviridiae).

Incomplete viruses, *see* defective viruses.

Infectious anemia virus of horses (unclassified). Particles of 90–140 nm width with 50 nm cores; buoyant density 1.18 g/ml in CsCl; ether sensitive; contains RNA. (Nakajima *et al.,* 1970.)

Infectious arteritis virus of horses, *see* equine arteritis virus.

Infectious bovine keratoconjunctivitis virus, infectious bovine rhino-tracheitis virus (bovine herpesvirus X and 1). Serologically related to human herpesviruses, but not by DNA homology. The buoyant density of the DNA in CsCl is 1.730 g/ml. (Graham *et al.,* 1972.)

Infectious bronchitis virus of chickens (coronavirus). Particles of 70–120 nm diameter, density 1.15 g/ml, ether sensitive. Surface carries characteristic projections. The nucleocapsid is probably loosely helical (8 nm diameter). (Cunningham *et al.,* 1972.)

Infectious canine hepatitis and laryngotracheitis viruses (adenoviruses).

Infectious hematopoietic necrosis virus of salmon (rhabdovirus). (Bachmann and Ahne, 1973.)

Infectious laryngotracheitis virus of chickens (phasianid herpesvirus 1). 45% (G+C). (Lee *et al.*, 1972.)

Infectious pancreatic necrosis virus of trout (as yet unclassified; possibly a diplornavirus). Hexagonal particles of 60–74 nm diameter, lacking inner capsid structure. Density of particle 1.33 g/ml in CsCl. The virus contains double-stranded RNA of 14 S, three components of 2.55–2.85 $\times$ 10^6 daltons. The three proteins (3%, 68%, and 29%) are of 80, 50, and 30 $\times$ 10^3 daltons. (Kelly and Loh, 1972.)

Influenza viruses (orthomyxovirus) (*see also* under myxoviruses). Type A, of man, swine, horse, duck, chicken; B of man; C of man. The three subtypes of A (formerly WSN, Lee strain, etc.) are now termed A0, A1, and A2. Minor cross reactions exist between A0 and A1 hemagglutinins and neuraminidases. Particles not uniform in shape (pleomorphic), 100 nm diameter spheres predominating, about 300 $\times$ 10^6 daltons in particle weight. Filamentous forms also exist, up to 4 μm long. The approximate composition of the virion is 66% protein, 25% lipid, 8% carbohydrate, and 0.9% RNA.

Particles consist of an outer membrane or envelope with projections or spikes, and an internal flexible rod or thread-shaped nucleocapsid. The envelope is 7–10 nm thick, the regularly spaced spikes 8–10 nm long and 7–9 nm apart (about 2000 per virion). Ether disrupts the envelope, releasing the nucleocapsid threads (50 to 130 nm long, with a 1 nm axial channel and of varying lengths) (see Electron micrograph VI).

The total RNA of each virion (38 S, 3–3.9 $\times$ 10^6, though according to more recent estimates 5.0 $\times$ 10^6 daltons) is present as probably 7 molecules of varying but definite sizes, combined but not covered with capsid protein, the RNA being nuclease-sensitive, the protein relatively protease-resistant. Isolated nucleocapsids show, among others, two peaks at 56 S and 64 S containing mainly 15 S RNA and 18 S RNA respectively. The lengths of the nucleocapsids range from 20 to 110 nm (three size groups).

The average composition is A/G/U/C = 22/20/36/23. The RNA chains start (5′) with ppp-A- and terminate mostly with 3′-unphosphorylated-U (doubtful). Differences in nucleotide sequences have been demonstrated between different RNA size groups.

The capsid (10% RNA, 90% protein) consists of two proteins,

one of a molecular weight of 53,000, 60,000, or 65,000 in different strains, or more likely in the hands of different investigators (about 1200 per particle), and another protein of 22,000–27,000 in equal to threefold quantity. It appears possible that the smaller represents the separate peptide chains and the larger a still disulfide-linked dimer. There also exist small amounts of two other larger proteins (80,000–90,000).

The envelope, including the spikes, consists largely of two biologically active proteins, the neuraminidase and the hemagglutinin, 10.8 S and 8.1 S, respectively. The neuraminidase consists of four identical glycopeptide chains, disulfide-linked in pairs, of about 63,000 mol. wt., and the hemagglutinin of two types of glycopeptide chains, of about 57,000 and 28,000 mol. wt., which are connected by disulfide bridges.

Influenza virus contains also an RNA polymerase.

For the amino acid composition of polypeptides isolated from influenza viruses, see Table 1. (Klenk *et al.*, 1972; Schulze, 1972; Laver and Baker, 1972.)

Inkoo virus (Bunyamwera supergroup). (Saikku *et al.*, 1971.)

INSECT VIRUSES. Viruses of almost all groups occurring in animals have been found in insects. Frequently insect viruses occur in large polyhedral inclusion bodies, and two large classes of occluded viruses have been distinguished, the cytoplasmic polyhedrosis viruses and the nuclear polyhedrosis viruses. The granulosis viruses are very similar to the latter; *see* under these listings.

Insect poxviruses. One originally isolated from larvae of the moth, *Amsacta,* grows on saltmarsh caterpillar. Many similar viruses have been found in beetles and other moths. 450 × 250 nm oval-shaped particle, in all detail similar to vaccinia (*see* melothonta poxvirus).

IRIDOVIRUS GROUP. Very large icosahedral DNA viruses, largely of insects. Tipula iridescent, sericestis iridescent, and chilo iridescent viruses, as well as possibly some frog viruses, African swinefever virus, Gecko virus, and lymphocystis virus of fish are members of the iridoviruses. The latter, in contrast to the insect iridoviruses, may be enveloped. All replicate in the cytoplasm (see Electron micrograph V).

Irituia virus (orbivirus subgroup of reoviridiae).

Israel turkey meningoencephalitis virus (flavivirus subgroup of togaviridiae).

Jaagsiekte virus, *see* sheep pulmonary adenomatosis virus.

Japanese B encephalitis virus (flavivirus subgroup of togaviridiae). One glycoprotein (lipoprotein?) of 53,000 mol. wt. and two proteins of 13,500 (the nucleocapsid protein) and 8700. (Shapiro *et al.*, 1971.)

JC virus (human polyoma virus related to SV-40). Probably associated with progressive multifocal leucoencephalopathy (PML). The disease but not the virus shows similarity to slow virus diseases.

Junin virus (arenavirus).

Junoniavirus (insect parvovirus related to *Galleria* densonucleosis virus).

K-virus of rats and mice (polyomavirus). Isometric particles of about 45 nm diameter. Capable of transforming mouse cells *in vitro*.

KBSH-virus (parvovirus). Particles of 20 nm diameter, 105 S, 5.3 × 10^6 particle weight, density in CsCl 1.395 g/ml. The virus contains 26.5% of 24 S single-stranded DNA (18 S in alkali), 1.4 or more probably 1.7 × 10^6 in molecular weight, density 1.724 g/ml. (Siegl *et al.*, 1971.)

Kemerovo virus (orbivirus subgroup of reoviridiae). Serologically unrelated to others.

Kern Canyon virus (rhabdovirus of myotis bats). Bullet-shaped particles of 73 × 132 nm containing three major structural proteins, of which the glycoprotein and the nucleocapsid protein (G and N) carry phosphate groups. The virion contains a protein kinase. Its proteins are similar to those of other rhabdoviruses. (Murphy and Fields, 1967; Sokol and Clark, 1973.)

Kilham rat virus (parvovirus). Isometric particles of 28 nm diameter, 6.6 × 10^6 particle weight (122 S), 1.43 g/ml density in CsCl (DNA lacking "top component" 1.32 g/ml); contains 27% of single-stranded linear DNA of buoyant density 1.715 in CsCl (16 S). The DNA of 1.6 × 10^6 mol. wt. is about 1500 nm long. A/G/T/C = 27/21/30/23. There are three major proteins, of 72, 62, and 55 × 10^3 daltons. The 62,000 mol. wt. protein represents 75% and is regarded as the capsid protein.

Kirk virus (rat parvovirus).

Kirsten virus, *see* murine leukemia virus.

Klamath virus (rhabdovirus of mice). 80 × 167 nm bullet-shaped particles.

Kokobera virus (flavivirus subgroup of togaviridiae).

Kunjin virus (flavivirus subgroup of togaviridiae). The 200 S particles, 48 nm in diameter, yield 143 S cores upon deoxycholate treatment, the same as for Sindbis virus cores (alphavirus subgroup). The RNA (38 S) of 4.2 × 10^6 daltons is said to disaggregate to half in 8 M urea (but newer data disagree with this interpretation). The major nucleocapsid protein is of 30,000 or 13,500 daltons, the envelope protein of 52,000 mol. wt. (earlier report: two smaller nucleocapsid proteins, adding up to 31,000). (Boulton and Westaway, 1972.)

Kuru disease agent of man, *see* slow viruses, scrapie.

Kyasanur Forest virus (flavivirus subgroup of togaviridiae). Affects man.

LaCrosse virus (member of California encephalitis virus group). Enveloped particle of 98 nm diameter with electron-dense core. Contains single-stranded RNA of six molecular weights, the larger of which dissociate upon heating. Three proteins were detected, of 85, 45, and 26 × 10^3 mol. wt. (McLerran and Arlinghaus, 1973.)

Lactic dehydrogenase (elevating) (Riley) virus of mice (probably togavirus). 235 S elliptical particles (about 47–56 nm); buoyant density in CsCl 1.12 g/ml; ether sensitive. Infective RNA of 5–6 × 10^6 daltons (48 S). The nucleocapsid protein is of 13,000, the envelope proteins 17,000 and 28,000 daltons, the latter only containing glucosamine. (Darnell and Plagemann, 1972.)

Lagos virus (rhabdovirus of bats, serologically related to rabies virus).

Lake Victoria cormorant virus (fowl herpesvirus) (Lee *et al.*, 1972.)

Langat virus (flavivirus subgroup of togaviridiae).

Laryngotracheitis virus (canine adenovirus).

Lassa (fever) virus (arenavirus).

Latent rat virus, *see* Kilham rat virus.

Latino virus (arenavirus).

LCV, L-cell virions (defective oncornaviruses). (Nichols *et al.*, 1973.)

Lebombo virus (orbivirus subgroup of reoviridiae).

LEUKOVIRUSES. The approved name for the group also called RNA-tumor viruses, which, however, has not gained general acceptance. The author prefers oncornaviruses and likes best the term retraviruses (for reverse transcriptase).*See* under oncornavirus group for description and members.

LK virus (equine herpesvirus). DNA of 84×10^6 daltons.

L-S virus (rat parvovirus).

Louping ill virus (flavivirus subgroup of togaviridiae). Causes a disease of sheep and cattle.

Lucké (frog adenocarcinoma) virus (ranid herpesvirus 1). A malignant, usually lethal frog tumor virus; contains DNA of 45% (G+C). (Granoff, 1972.)

Lumpy skin disease virus (cattlepox virus).

Lu III (parvovirus). Similar properties to, though serologically distinguishable from, KBSH virus.

Lymphocystis (tumor) virus, from the Atlantic croaker (icosahedral cytoplasmic DNA virus, possibly a member of iridovirus group or a herpesvirus?). 200–600 nm icosahedral particles, enveloped, with long attached filaments, ether sensitive. Probably DNA containing. Causes chronic disease and tumors in many fishes. (Zwillenberg and Wolf, 1968.)

Lymphocytic choriomeningitis virus (prototype of arenaviruses). Variable-size particles (about 120 nm in diameter containing several 20–30 nm diameter electron-dense granules. Density in CsCl 1.18 g/ml, about 500 S; contains seven single-stranded RNA species, of which two (23 S and 31 S) are virus-specific. The others may be from ribosomes which may represent the typical intraviral granules. Various light disease symptoms in many mammals. (Welsh *et al.,* 1972; Pedersen, 1973.)

M9 virus (orbivirus subgroup of reoviridiae).

M25 virus, *see* parainfluenza virus type 4.

Machupo virus (arenavirus).

Maedi virus of sheep (slow virus, related to Visna virus). Shows many similarities to oncornaviruses; contains 62 S, 35 S, and 13 S RNA as well as reverse transcriptase and DNA-dependent DNA polymerase. (Lin and Thormar, 1972.)

Malignant catarrh virus of cattle (herpesvirus).

Mammary tumor viruses, *see* mouse mammary tumor virus.

Marburg virus (rhabdovirus). Variably long (130 to 1200 nm, mean length 665 nm × 80 nm) particles, often sharply bent. Simian (and human) pathogen. (Siegert, 1972.)

Marek's disease virus (phasianid herpesvirus 2). Double-stranded DNA, 56 S, 120×10^6 mol. wt. (in alkali 70 S, 60×10^6); density 1.705 g/ml; 46% (G+C). The protein pattern is similar to that of herpes simplex and pseudorabies virus. The virus shows serological relationship with common herpesvirus. Oncogenic in chickens, now controlled by vaccines. (Chen *et al.,* 1972.)

Mason-Pfizer monkey virus (unclassified oncornavirus). Buoyant density 1.155 g/ml in CsCl. Contains RNA of 70×10^6 daltons. (Manning and Hackett, 1972.)

Mayaro virus (alphavirus subgroup of togaviridiae). Contains two proteins.

MC-29 virus (avian leukosis virus).

ME virus, *see* mouse-Elberfeld virus.

Measles virus of man (paramyxovirus). Closely related to canine distemper virus and rinderpest virus of cattle. 150 nm particles of buoyant density in CsCl of about 1.27 g/ml. Contains helical nucleocapsid of about 17 × 1100 nm, 6 nm pitch, 11–13 protein subunits per turn (280 S). The RNA in the nucleocapsids (5%) is resistant to pancreatic ribonuclease.

The RNA of 52 S has a molecular weight of 6.4×10^6 daltons. The nucleocapsid protein has a molecular weight of 60,000. The virion contains five additional proteins of 76, 69, 53, 51, and 46 × 10^3 mol. wt., which are identical to those of canine distemper virus.

Measles virus hemagglutinates only primate erythrocytes and lacks neuraminidase, thus hemagglutinating optimally at elevated temperature. (Schluederberg, 1971; Hall and Martin, 1973.)

Melothonta (insect) poxvirus (occluded). Oval 400 × 250 nm particles resembling poxviruses in all respects; *see also* under insect poxviruses. (Bergoin *et al.,* 1971.)

Mengo virus (cardiovirus subgroup of picornaviridiae). 28 nm particles, 151 S, 8.5 × 10⁶ particle weight (*see* mouse-Elberfeld virus for capsid architecture). 31% RNA, 2.6 × 10⁶ mol. wt.; A/G/U/C = 26/23/26/25. Proteins: 34,000, 30,500, 24,000, and 7300 (plus a minor component of 40,000) mol. wt. (probably equimolar amounts; *see* mouse-Elberfeld virus). (Miller and Plagemann, 1972.)

Middleburg virus (alphavirus subgroup of togaviridiae).

Milker's nodule virus (pseudocowpox) (paravaccinia subgroup of poxvirus).

Mink enteritis virus (probably a parvovirus).

Minute virus of mice (MVM) (parvovirus). 20–25 nm diameter, 1.42 g/ml density. Contains single-stranded DNA, 1.72 g/ml density in CsCl, 1.7 × 10⁶ mol. wt., A/G/T/C = 27/19/33/21. (Tattersall, 1972.)

MM virus (cardiovirus subgroup of picornaviridiae).

Modoc virus (flavivirus subgroup of togaviridiae).

Molluscum contagiosum virus of man (poxvirus). Similar to vaccinia in DNA content (density 1.288 g/ml, vaccinia 1.287 g/ml, 5250 S *vs.* 5150 S). Oncogenic. (Pirie *et al.*, 1971.)

Moloney murine leukemia virus, *see* murine leukemia virus.

Monkeypox virus (vaccinia subgroup of poxviruses). The DNA has a molecular weight of 159 × 10⁶ and 38% (G+C). (Yau and Rouhandeh, 1973.)

Mono Lake virus (orbivirus subgroup of reoviridiae).

Montana myotis leukoencephalitis virus (flavivirus subgroup of togaviridiae).

Mosquito iridescent virus (iridovirus). Two strains (*R*MIV and *T*MIV) which are serologically identical but differ in size and sedimentation rate. Isoelectric points pH 3.15 and 3.30. The 260/280 nm ratios are 1.20 and 1.21, and A_{max} (0.1%) is 6.32 and 5.47, the diameters about 185 and 210 nm, the densities in CsCl 1.32 and 1.31 g/ml, the sedimentation coefficients 4041 and 3318 S, and the particle weights 2.75 and 2.1 × 10⁹ daltons. (Wagner *et al.*, 1973; Stoltz and Summers, 1972.)

Mount Elgon virus (rhabdovirus of bats and mosquitos). Bullet-shaped in tissue, 226 × 688 nm. (Murphy *et al.*, 1970a.)

Mouse-Elberfeld (ME) virus (cardiovirus subgroup of picornaviridiae). Virions of 24 nm diameter, 8.4×10^6 particle weight, 155 S. The nucleocapsid consists of 31% single-stranded RNA, molecular weight 2.6×10^6, A/G/U/C = 25/24/27/24, and four proteins in equimolar amounts, 33,000 (α), 30,500 (β), 25,800 (γ), 7300 (δ), and varying small amounts of a 41,000 (ϵ) species (composed of β + δ). The architectural principle of the picornavirus capsids consisting of four and at times five proteins was first established with this virus. It appears that both ($\epsilon + \alpha + \gamma$) and ($\alpha + \beta + \gamma + \delta$) add up to 96,000 in molecular weight. Since it is now well established for many picornaviruses, particularly poliomyelitis virus, that a large precursor protein is split in a specific manner, in part prior to capsid assembly and in part during virus maturation, it appears that all these capsids are built up as regular icosahedral arrays of 60 units composed of three (ϵ,α,γ) or, after the final proteolytic step, four peptide chains ($\alpha,\beta,\gamma,\delta$). For the amino acid composition of the polypeptide components of encephalomyocarditis and mouse-Elberfeld viruses, see Table 1. (Stoltzfus and Rueckert, 1972.)

Mouse hepatitis virus (coronavirus).

Mouse leukemia virus, *see* murine leukemia virus.

Mouse mammary tumor virus (Bittner virus, B-type particles) (oncornavirus). Density of whole virus 1.17, nucleoid 1.24 g/ml. RNA content: whole virus, 1.9, nucleoid 4.4%. The envelope shows a smooth surface membrane, in contrast to C-type particles. The dense centrally located nucleoid contains nucleocapsid strands of 8–9 nm diameter containing S1 and S2, group-specific antigens. The S3–S5, type-specific antigens, are located in the envelope; all are synthesized in the cytoplasm. Proteins: 90,000, 70,000, 52,000 (the major nucleoid, S1), 33,000, 23,000 (the major membrane proteins, S3). (Sarkar *et al.*, 1971; Nowinski *et al.*, 1971.)

Mouse polyoma virus, *see* polyoma virus.

MP tumor virus (unclassified) (Molomut *et al.*, 1964.)

MP 359, MRM 10434 (orbivirus subgroup of reoviridiae).

Mucambo virus (alphavirus subgroup of togaviridiae).

Mumps virus (parainfluenza subgroup of paramyxoviruses). 150 nm diameter particles, containing an 1100 nm stretched-out nucleocapsid in helix of 6 nm pitch, about 12 protein subunits/turn. The RNA is of 50 S. The virus contains neuraminidase. (East and Kingsbury, 1972.)

Murine encephalomyelitis virus (picornavirus).

Murine hepatitis virus (coronavirus).

Murine leukemia virus (Rauscher, Friend, Moloney, Gross, Kirsten, Harvey viruses, etc.) (transformation-defective C-type oncornaviruses). Approximately spherical, enveloped particles, 106 nm in diameter upon freeze drying and negative staining, with 8 nm diameter weakly bound surface knobs. The core of 80 nm diameter of icosahedral symmetry consists of 6 nm subunits, 7.5 nm apart. The virions are of 1.18 g/ml density in CsCl, the cores (representing about 25%) of 1.226 g/ml density. There also can be seen one or two envelope membranes, 12 and 20 nm thick. The single-stranded RNA has been stated to be homogeneous after heating (although others report the presence of an 18 S component of different composition), 38 S, of about 3.8×10^6 mol. wt., it contains A-rich sequences. Among the five main proteins are the group-specifc (capsid) antigen of 31×10^3, a glycoprotein of 86, and proteins of 15, 12, and 10×10^3 daltons. Among various enzymes there is reverse transcriptase. (Moroni, 1972; Schäfer *et al.*, 1972.)

Murine sarcoma virus (replication-defective oncornavirus). Moloney and Harvey strains produce tumors in hamsters. The protein pattern of Harvey sarcoma virus is very similar to that of the Rauscher leukemia virus. (Moroni, 1972.)

Murray Valley encephalitis virus (flavivirus subgroup of togaviridiae).

Myxoma viruses, subgroup of poxviruses, mostly of rabbits and related species. Largely oncogenic.

MYXOVIRUS GROUP (also called orthomyxoviruses. Members: influenza viruses types A [human, porcine, equine, and avian viruses] and B and C [only human types known]). Large (100 nm diameter), somewhat pleomorphic enveloped particles containing multiple chains of single-stranded RNA in helical nucleocapsids (about 6 [A,B] or 9 [C] nm in diameter) (see Electron micrograph VI). Sensitive to lipid solvents. Buoyant density in sucrose about 1.20

for A, B, and 1.18 for C. RNA synthesized in the nucleus, the envelope during passage through the plasma membrane. Filamentous forms also exist. Virions contain RNA polymerase. The envelopes carry spikes consisting of neuraminidase and hemagglutinin. Their lipid compositions reflect those of the plasma membrane of the host cell, except for the absence of neuraminic acid in the lipids—probably a consequence of the presence of the neuraminidase (*see* influenza virus).

Nariva virus (rodent paramyxovirus, unrelated to other known groups).

Ndumu virus (alphavirus subgroup of togaviridiae).

Nebraska calf diarrhea virus (reovirus).

Negishi virus (flavivirus subgroup of togaviridiae).

Nelson Bay virus (reovirus).

Newcastle disease virus (paramyxovirus of chickens). Roughly spherical, about 200 nm diameter, 500×10^6 dalton particle weight. The buoyant density in CsCl varies from 1.212 to 1.242. The spikes are less prominent than in influenza virus (8 nm long, 1.5 nm diameter, 8–10 nm apart). The helical nucleocapsid is about 1000 nm long and 18 nm in diameter. The virion consists of 67% protein, 24% liquid, 7% carbohydrate, and 1% RNA.

The single-stranded RNA is probably about 6×10^6 in molecular weight (56 S). The composition is $A/G/U/C = 24/24/29/23$.

The main envelope glycoproteins are 9.3 S and 6.1 S; the larger carries both the hemagglutinin and the neuraminidase activity (as is the case for other paramyxoviruses). They consist of peptide chains of 74 and 56×10^3 daltons. The main capsid protein (45%) is 56×10^3 and a membrane protein 41×10^3 daltons. Yield per cell: 0.1 PFU in mouse kidney cells to 100 in CV-1 monkey kidney cells. (Scheid and Choppin, 1973.)

Nodamura virus (insect picornavirus). 28 nm particle (140 S) of density in CsCl of 1.34 g/ml. Said to contain two RNAs of 22 S and 15 S (molecular weights 1 and 0.5×10^6), $A/G/U/C = 22/28/23/27$ and $25/23/24/28$ respectively, and only one major protein of 46,000 daltons. Host and vector *Culex tritaeniorhynchus,* a mosquito; also a vertebrate, possibly swine. This appears to be the only animal covirus known (see page 76), the two RNA's being only cooperatively infectious. (Murphy *et al.,* 1970b; Brown and Hull, 1973.)

Ntaya virus (flavivirus subgroup of togaviridiae).

Nuclear polyhedrosis viruses of insects, usually from silkworm (members of baculovirus group of rod-shaped occluded insect viruses). Virions are embedded in membrane-covered "crystalline" inclusion bodies of 0.5–15 μm ("polyhedra"). This matrix consists largely of 11 S protein. The rod-shaped virions are of complex structure, frequently with terminal protrusions, 40–70 $\times$ 250–400 nm, covered with a membrane and containing a dense core. The virions are sensitive to ether. They contain double-stranded DNA, predominantly of 80 $\times$ 10^6 mol. wt. but ranging from 59 $\times$ 10^6 to 118 $\times$ 10^6, with contour lengths from 30 to 60 nm, partly linear and partly open circular. The composition is 37–59% (G+C). They replicate in the nucleus. The silkworm (*Bombyx mori*) nuclear polyhedrosis virus (80 $\times$ 330 nm rods) contains 8% DNA of 13.1 S, 41% (G+C). The isolated DNA is infectious. (Harrap, 1972.)

O-agent from cattle and sheep (orbivirus). Structurally indistinguishable from SA 11 virus, though serologically these are unrelated.

OC-43 (prototype coronavirus).

Omsk hemorraghic fever virus of man (flavivirus subgroup of togaviridiae).

ONCORNAVIRUS GROUP. Not yet officially accepted term for leukoviruses or RNA tumor viruses, all equally imperfect names.* Medium large (100 nm diameter) enveloped and ether-sensitive particles; studded in regular manner with projections and containing a dense eccentric nucleoid. The 60–70 S RNA (1.5%), of 10–12 $\times$ 10^6 daltons, dissociates with heat, DMSO, etc., to 30–35 S and smaller single-stranded RNA (10 S, 8 S, 7 S, 4 S, etc.). The partly helical nucleocapsids are 7–9 nm in diameter.

All oncornaviruses contain RNA-dependent DNA polymerase (= reverse transcriptase), also active as ribonuclease H which degrades only DNA-bound (= hybridized) RNA. Also other polymerases, nucleases, and many other enzymes occur in these viruses. The general protein pattern shows at least seven proteins of molecular weights 100,000, 70,000, 29,000, 19,000 (only in avian oncornaviruses), 15,000, 12,000, and 10,000. (For more detail, *see* under individual oncornaviruses.)

Members of the RNA tumor virus group are (A) Rous and other fowl viruses; RAV and RIF viruses; RPL 12; avian leucosis

* New proposal: retraviruses (for reverse transcriptase containing).

and myeloblastosis (AMV) viruses; osteopetrosis virus; Fujinami sarcoma virus, FAV-1; (B) murine leukemia and sarcoma viruses (Gross, Friend, Graffi, Moloney, Rauscher, etc.); (C) feline leukemia and sarcoma viruses; (D) mouse mammary tumor virus (Bittner) and nodule-inducing virus; (E) reticuloendotheliosis virus. All but (D) are also called C-type particles.

O'Nyong-nyong virus (alphavirus subgroup of togaviridiae).

ORBIVIRUSES (one of two subgroups of reoviridiae). Prototype: bluetongue virus. These are somewhat smaller than the reoviruses and more sensitive to low pH. They are slightly sensitive to ether. The surface architecture of the orbiviruses also differs from that of the reoviruses in that they may consist of a single shell of 32 capsomeres. However, the differences between orbiviruses and typical reoviruses are diminishing as more is being learned about them. These viruses, previously ungrouped or in minor serogroups, include bluetongue, epizootic hemorrhagic disease of deer, Eubenangee, IbAr 22619, B 1327, Colorado tick fever, African horse sickness, Irituia, Changuinola, BeAr 35646, BeAr 41067, Kemerovo, Chenuda, Tribec, Wad Medani, Mono Lake, Huacho, Lebombo, Palyam, D'Aguilar, G 8886, G 15534, Corriparta, Acado, MP 359, CH 9935, and MRM 10434 viruses. (Borden *et al.,* 1971; Murphy *et al.,* 1971).

Oregon sockeye disease virus (rhabdovirus of salmon).

Orf virus (contagious pustular dermatitis virus, "contagious ecthyma," paravaccinia subgroup of poxvirus). Infects sheep and goats (also man). Particles about 250 × 160 nm; nucleoprotein threads (7–9 nm) form characteristic lattice in transparent matrix. Some subtypes are enveloped and ether sensitive. Orf virus is antigenically as well as morphologically related to poxviruses.

Orteca virus, related to yaba and tanapox viruses.

Orthomyxoviruses, *see* myxoviruses.

Osteopetrosis virus (avian leukosis virus).

Owl herpesvirus (Lee *et al.,* 1972.)

P-virus of *Drosophila melanogaster* (picornavirus). About 27 nm in diameter. Symptomless. (Teninges and Plus, 1972.)

Palyam virus (orbivirus subgroup of reoviridiae).

Papilloma viruses (the larger-sized subgroup of papovaviridiae, including bovine, canine, human, rabbit papilloma, i.e., Shope rabbit papilloma virus, etc.). Generally cause benign warts, rarely cause transformation in tissue culture ($1/10^9$ for human, possibly $1/10^5$ for bovine papilloma virus) or cytopathic effects. Particles are of 53 nm diameter, 290 S, 47×10^6 dalton particle weight. The virion is of skew icosahedral structure, $T = 7$, 72 capsomeres (420 polypeptide chains, 60 hexamers, 12 pentamers) (see Electron micrograph VII). Contains 12% cyclic double-stranded DNA, 5×10^6 mol. wt. (density 1.711 g/ml); (G+C) content 41, 43, 46, and 47% for human, canine, bovine, and Shope rabbit papilloma virus DNA. The DNA has two sedimentation constants, due to its circular state, in part supercoiled, and in part relaxed through at least one break in one strand. Linear molecules, the result of both strands being broken near one another, also exist. (Klug and Finch, 1968.)

PAPOVAVIRIDIAE. Family of viruses including the *pa*pilloma and *po*lyoma viruses, and *va*cuolating agent, i.e., SV-40. Medium small viruses of cubic symmetry (about 50 nm) containing double-stranded cyclic DNA of molecular weight $3-5 \times 10^6$. These viruses replicate in the nucleus; many of them are oncogenic.

PARAINFLUENZA VIRUSES (subgroup of paramyxoviruses). Four serotypes: (1) hemadsorption virus 2 (man); Sendai virus (mouse, pig, man?); (2) croup-associated virus (man); SV-5, SV-41 (monkey); (3) hemadsorption virus 1 (man); shipping fever virus (cattle), respiratory equine virus; (4) M25 (man), mumps virus. For structural detail, *see* SV-5, Sendai virus, etc.

Paralysis virus of termites (picornavirus). About 25 nm in diameter. Symptomless.

PARAMYXOVIRUS GROUP. Virions similar but larger (about 150 nm diameter, 700×10^6 particle weight) than those of myxoviruses. Contain about 1% of a single molecule of $6-7 \times 10^6$ single-stranded RNA (56 S) in a helical 18-nm-diameter, 1000-nm-long nucleocapsid, very similar in appearance to tobacco mosaic virus. The envelopes are similar to those of myxoviruses in structure, appearance, and origin (see Electron micrograph VIII). The viruses are ether sensitive. All paramyxoviruses hemagglutinate, but some (e.g., measles virus) lack the neuraminidase, a characteristic feature of all myxoviruses and many paramyxoviruses. Most paramyxoviruses cause fusion of host cells (polykaryons) at high multiplicity of infection. Main members (all serologically interrelated): parainfluenza viruses 1–4, Newcastle disease virus, mumps virus. Measles, distemper, and rinderpest viruses represent a subgroup. The RNA of paramyxovirions, as those of rhabdo- and probably myxoviruses, represents the complement to the messenger strand; the term "negative strand" has been proposed.

Parana virus (arenavirus).

Parvovirus group (small DNA viruses; logical but not accepted name: picodnaviruses, analogous to picorna, small RNA viruses). Small, 18–22 nm diameter, icosahedral particles (buoyant density in CsCl 1.38–1.45 g/ml). The virion consists of probably 32 capsomeres of 2–4 nm diameter. They contain 18–34% single-stranded DNA of $1.2–2.1 \times 10^6$ daltons which in some are both of the complementary strands; then isolated DNA tends to anneal and appear double-stranded. Parvoviruses are partly infective (MVM, Kilham rat virus, etc.), partly defective and thus requiring infection by a helper virus (adeno-associated viruses). The viruses replicate in the nucleus; they are quite heat stable; several of them hemagglutinate widely.

Some certain or probable members of the parvoviruses are: H 1–3 and X-14 viruses, latent rat (Kilham) virus, minute mouse virus, porcine, bovine, and avian parvoviruses, densonucleosis and Junonia virus, mink enteritis, hemorrhagic encephalopathy, feline panleucopenia, and the defective adeno-associated viruses. (Tinsley and Longworth, 1973.)

Pichinde virus (arenavirus). The multiple single-stranded RNA species are probably in part from ribosomes (*see* lymphocytic choriomeningitis virus). The virus contains four proteins (two of 72,000, one of 34,000, and a minor component of 12,000 mol. wt. The second and third are glycoproteins). (Carter *et al.,* 1973.)

Picodnaviruses, *see* parvovirus group.

Picornaviridiae. Large family of small RNA viruses characterized by icosahedral particles (25–30 nm diameter) consisting of usually four proteins forming sixty equal capsomeres and one molecule of RNA of 2.6×10^6 mol. wt. Both RNA and protein are replicated in the cytoplasm. The protein is split to form the four components amounting to 96,000 daltons (molecular weights about 35,000, 30,000, 24,000, and 7000), partly during assembly. The virions contain no enzymes. The RNA serving directly as messenger carries 3'-terminal poly(A). Subgroups are the enteroviruses, cardioviruses, rhinoviruses, and foot and mouth disease virus (*see* poliomyelitis, encephalomyocarditis (EMC), mouse-Elberfeld (ME) virus, etc.). In a broader sense most plant and many bacterial viruses are picornaviruses (small RNA viruses), although these usually consist of only one or two proteins forming the icosahedral 20–30 nm nucleocapsid with usually one molecule of RNA of up to 2×10^6 daltons. (Brown and Hull, 1973.)

Pig enteroviruses (picornavirus). Ten serotypes (e.g., Talfan, Teschen, F43, etc.); 28 nm diameter particles.

Pigeonpox virus (birdpox subgroup of poxviruses).

Pistillo virus (arenavirus).

Pixuna virus (alphavirus subgroup of togaviridiae).

PML-2 agent, *see* JC virus.

Pneumonia virus of mice ("meta" myxovirus, similar to respiratory syncytial viruses).

Pneumotropic virus (coronavirus of rats).

Poliomyelitis virus (enterovirus subgroup of picornaviridiae). Three serotypes are known. Poliovirus is infectious only in primates. Its icosahedral particles have a 28 nm diameter; 158 S; density 1.34 g/ml; particle weight probably 8.4×10^6. Virion contains 31% single-stranded RNA, 2.4×10^6 mol. wt. (2300 nm long?), $A/G/U/C = 30/23/24/23$. The RNA contains a 3'-terminal poly(A) sequence of about 89 adenylic acid residues, preceded by two guanylic acid residues, and 5'-terminal pA-. Proteins: 35,000 IV; 29,000 II; 25,000 III; 7300 I (and minor components of about 30,000). (Formerly reported percentages and molar ratios are probably erroneous.) Actually, by analogy to mouse-Elberfeld virus, mature poliomyelitis probably consists of four equimolar protein components. N-terminal are aspartic acid, glycine, and serine. (The roman numbers above indicate gene-map order, 5' to 3'). (Tannock *et al.,* 1970; Phillips, 1972.)

Polyhedral cytoplasmic DNA virus, *see* frog virus 3.

Polyhedrosis viruses, *see* cytoplasmic and nuclear polyhedrosis viruses.

Polyoma viruses (the smaller-sized subgroup of papovaviridiae, including polyoma virus, SV-40, rabbit kidney vacuolating virus, etc.). Icosahedral particles ($T = 7$) of 45 nm diameter, 240 S, particle weight 28×10^6. Density of virion in CsCl 1.34 g/ml; of empty protein-only particles 1.29 g/ml (see Electron micrograph IX). Virus contains 12% of double-stranded DNA, 2.8×10^6 mol. wt., density 1.709 g/ml, 48% (G+C). The DNA is circular and consists of two or three density components due to the presence of hypercoiled (20.3 S) and relaxed circles caused by at least one break in one strand (15.8 S). Linear molecules, due to vicinal breaks of both strands, are 14.4 S (these also probably represent linear host DNA from pseudovirions).

The main protein (about 60%) has a molecular weight of 48,000; three others are 86,000, 35,000, and 23,000. Three small proteins (15,000–19,000) represent host cell histones. The architecture of the polyoma virus is still in dispute, with 72, 42, and 32 capsomeres being considered. The viruses are assembled in the nucleus. The polyoma virus is lytic in mouse cells and temperate, causing transformations, in hamster and rat cells (30–100 particles produce a plaque); compared to other DNA viruses, it is relatively efficient in causing transformation of cells ($1/10^5$ particles); it can be oncogenic in animals. (Roblin *et al.*, 1971; Friedmann and David, 1972.)

Powassan virus (of man) (flavivirus subgroup of togaviridiae).

POXVIRUS GROUP. Very large brick-shaped particles (about 200×300 nm, 5000 S) containing about 6% of linear DNA of $160–200 \times 10^6$ mol. wt., 35–40% (G+C). The particles are of complex morphology, with several membranes, internal biconcave nucleoid or core, lateral bodies, etc. (see Electron micrograph X). The poxviruses are generally more or less ether resistant and relatively stable to heat and acid. They replicate in cytoplasmic "factories." The virions contain many proteins, including many enzymes, such as the DNA-dependent RNA polymerase associated with the core, as well as nucleases, ATPase, etc.

Poxviruses frequently produce no apparent disease. Several strains hemagglutinate. Six subgroups have been identified as occurring in most vertebrates, besides very similar viruses detected in insects (entomopoxviruses). The poxviruses which cause diseases in man, birds, and mammals, but not usually tumors, are often transmitted by insect vectors. (Andrewes and Pereira, 1972.)

Members of Subgroup I, related to variola, are: variola, alastrim, vaccinia, rabbitpox, monkeypox, ectromelia, cowpox, buffalopox.

Members of Subgroup II, related to orf virus, are: orf, milker's nodes (paravaccinia), bovine papular stomatitis.

Members of Subgroup III (other viruses affecting ungulates) are: sheeppox, goatpox, lumpy skin disease.

Members of Subgroup IV (avian poxes) are: fowlpox, canarypox, and other bird poxes.

Members of Subgroup V (viruses related to myxoma) are: rabbit myxoma, rabbit fibroma, hare fibroma, squirrel fibroma.

Members of Subgroup VI (unclassified poxviruses) are: molluscum contagiosum, swinepox, tanapox virus, yaba virus, horsepox, camelpox.

Prague virus (nondefective avian sarcoma virus).

Progressive multifocal leukoencephalopathy agent, see JC virus and SV-40.

Progressive pneumonitis virus (possibly the same as Maedi virus, a "slow" virus, seemingly related to oncornaviruses and specifically to Visna virus). Single-stranded 60–70 S RNA which becomes 35 S upon melting. Contains reverse transcriptase. (Stone *et al.*, 1972.)

Pseudocowpox virus (a poxvirus related to contagious pustular dermatitis virus).

Pseudorabies virus of swine (subgroup A herpesvirus). Related to herpes simplex virus, but lacking DNA sequence homology. The DNA is said to occur as two components of 26 S and 31 S [77% (G+C)]. The protein pattern is similar to that of Marek's disease virus. (Graham *et al.*, 1972.)

Pseudoviruses, *see* defective viruses.

Rabbit fibromavirus (myxoma-subgroup of poxviruses). Double-stranded DNA, 153×10^6 mol. wt., 40.4% (G+C), differs from vaccinia DNA, 35.5% (G+C). Oncogenic. (Jacquemont *et al.,* 1972.)

Rabbit kidney vacuolating virus (polyomavirus). The DNA of 2.8×10^6 mol. wt. is circular, partly hypercoiled, 43% (G+C).

Rabbit myxomavirus, *see* myxomavirus.

Rabbit (oral) papillomavirus, *see* Shope rabbit papillomavirus.

Rabbitpox virus (vaccinia subgroup of poxvirus).

Rabies virus of mammals (rhabdovirus). Bullet-shaped, 80×180 nm particles (600 S), with lipid-containing envelope. Virus matures largely in the plasma membrane, and its lipid composition resembles that of the membrane, with relatively high cholesterol and sphingolipid content. Virus loses some lipid during purification, its density increasing from 1.14 to 1.16 g/ml in the process. The 1000-nm-long nucleocapsid (200 S, 120 $\times$ 10^6 daltons) consists of 1300 protein subunits and single-stranded RNA (45 S), 4.6 $\times$ 10^6 mol. wt.; A/G/U/C = 26/21/29/23. The envelope and spikes (7 nm long) consist of three proteins, 1783 molecules of 80,000 mol. wt. glycoprotein (G), the protein forming the spikes; 789 molecules of 40,000; and 1661 of 25,000. The nucleocapsid consists of 1713 molecules of protein of 62,000 (N) and 76 of 55,000 mol. wt. (Nm). The N protein was found to be a phosphoprotein. The virus hemagglutinates best at low temperature. The virion contains a protein kinase but no neuraminidase. Rabies virus replicates in many mammals. (György *et al.*, 1971; Sokol and Clark, 1973.)

Rat virus (RV), *see* Kilham rat virus.

Rauscher murine leukemia virus (transformation-defective murine leukemia virus).

RAV 0, 1–7, 49, 50, 60 (Rous associated viruses) (transformation-defective avian leukosis viruses).

RD 114 virus (transformation-defective oncornavirus). C-type virus isolated from human tumor cells, but derivation from a feline virus appears more probable.

Red disease agent of pike (rhabdovirus). (Kinkelin *et al.*, 1973.)

REOVIRIDIAE. Proposed name for the double-stranded RNA-containing viruses of animals (reo- and orbiviruses), plants, and insects. Preferred name, at least for the plant and insect viruses: diplornaviruses. (*See* diplornavirus group.)

REOVIRUSES (one of two subgroups of the animal diplornaviruses) (*r*espiratory and *e*nteric *o*rphan viruses). First classified as echo virus 10. At least three serotypes are known.
    Reovirus particles, 630 S, 100 $\times$ 10^6 in particle weight, consist of inner and outer protein shells. The core is 52 nm in diameter, the complete particle 76 nm (see Electron micrograph IV). Particles lacking the outer shell occur naturally and can be obtained by chymotrypsin treatment of the larger virion; they are infectious. The capsomeres in the outer shell are of 9 nm diameter, those of

the inner shell 4 nm. Both shells appear to be of icosahedral symmetry, consisting of 92 or 122 capsomeres of different size, with the core carrying 12 projections halfway into the outer shell (10 nm in diameter). The RNA (15%) is double-stranded, 43% (G+C) on average, and occurs in ten distinct molecular species of molecular weights ranging from 2.4 to 0.6 $\times$ 10^6 daltons. All ten segments start (5′) with ppGp-pyrimidin and terminate (3′) with unphosphorylated cytidine. Oligonucleotides also occur in the virion, one group starting with pppG- of lengths up to 9, and another of oligo-A of 2–20 residues, starting with pppA-. Both groups also exist with only one or two 5′-terminal phosphates.

The proteins of type 3 reovirus (Dearing strain) were found to be of molecular weight 155,000 (λ1, 113 molecules); 140,000 (λ2, 80 molecules; the major surface protein of the core); 80,000 (μ1, 23 molecules); 72,000 (μ2, 550 molecules); 42,000 (σ1, 31 molecules); 38,000 (σ2, 202 molecules); and 34,000 (σ3, 890 molecules); (5000–10,000?, about 500 molecules). Proteins μ2 and σ3 are located on the surface of the virion. Enzyme treatment, removing the outer shell (and the A-rich RNA), leaves only the two largest and the 38,000 mol. wt. protein. For amino acid composition, see Table 1. The amino-terminal sequence of μ2 is Pro-Gly-Gly-Val-Pro-; all other proteins have blocked N-terminals. The C-terminal sequences of σ3 is (-(Val, Leu, Val)); those of μ2 and λ1 and λ2 are -Arg preceded by different amino acids.

The RNA remains nuclease resistant in the core. The virion contains a latent RNA polymerase activated by heating or chymotrypsin treatment and thus present in the core. This enzyme may serve first as transcriptase and release messenger RNA, and later it may replicate both strands.

Relation to any human disease uncertain, but pathogenic upon inoculation. Newborn mice seriously affected by reovirus type 3. Reoviruses have been found in man and other mammals as well as in birds and mosquitoes, but no evidence for their multiplication in insect vectors has been found. Reoviruses, widely distributed in nature, cause marked cytopathic effects in tissue culture. They are nonenveloped and are thus resistant to lipid solvents. They agglutinate human erythrocytes, their receptors, in contrast to those of myxo- and paramyxoviruses, not being susceptible to the receptor-destroying enzyme of *Vibrio cholerae*. (Joklik, 1972; Pett *et al.*, 1973.)

Reptilian C-type virus (oncornavirus). (Gilden *et al.*, 1970.)

Respiratory equine virus, *see* parainfluenza virus.

Respiratory syncytial virus (human and bovine) (not yet classified; "metamyxovirus"). 80–120 nm diameter particles, with projections and helical nucleocapsids of 11–15 nm diameter. Does not hemagglutinate. (Ito *et al.*, 1973b.)

Reticuloendotheliosis virus, similar in morphology but not biologically and serologically related to avian leukosis or sarcoma viruses. Buoyant density in CsCl 1.20 g/ml (Rous sarcoma virus 1.24). The properties of the RNA show similarities to those of AMV. At least three proteins of 30, 20, and 12×10^3 and two glycoproteins of 65 and 18×10^3 mol. wt. have been observed, differing in molecular weight from those of RAV. The virus contains reverse transcriptase (Maldonado and Bose, 1972, 1973.)

RHABDOVIRUS GROUP. Medium large though somewhat variable bullet-shaped particles (e.g., 70×200 nm, 200×10^6 dalton particle weight). Lipid-containing envelope and 10 nm spikes can be seen as well as at times two transverse striation patterns of different periodicity. At least one of these is due to the helical nucleocapsid enclosing the simple molecule of $3.5–4.5 \times 10^6$ dalton RNA (2%). These viruses contain RNA polymerase and the RNA is the negative strand and must first be transcribed. They are ether sensitive. Prototype: Vesicular stomatitis virus. Others are: Cocal, Flanders Hart Park, Kern Canyon, rabies, and probably Egtved, Gomphrena, Lagos bat, Mount Elgon bat virus, possibly Marburg virus. *Drosophila* sigma virus represents an insect rhabdovirus. Also many plant viruses are rhabdoviruses, although these appear generally to be at least partly bacilliform rather than bullet shaped. It is not certain whether either form should be regarded as an artefact. (See Electron micrograph XI.)

Rhinopneumonitis virus, *see* equine abortion virus.

RHINOVIRUS GROUP (subgroup of the picornaviridiae). More than 90 human serotypes known; also an equine and several bovine types (sd1, 181/v, C-07, EC11, RS 3X). There is little or no serological relationship or nucleotide sequence homology among the rhinoviruses. The human rhinoviruses are 22–28 nm particles of 158 S, 1.38–1.41 g/ml in density in CsCl (compared to enteroviruses 1.33–1.34 g/ml). Serotype 14 is of 25 nm diameter, 158 S (same as poliovirus), 7.1 (or more probably 8.4) $\times 10^6$ particle weight. The 260/280 absorbance ratio is about 1.71. The viruses contain 29.8%

(28 S) RNA of probable molecular weight 2.6×10^6 (same as poliovirus). The HGP strain is reported as 22 nm in diameter, 150 S. $A/G/U/C = 34/20/26/20$. The proteins are similar to those of other picornaviruses in molecular weight, all four occurring in equimolar proportion (34,000, 30,000, 26,000, 7000). *See* mouse-Elberfeld virus for architecture of picornaviruses. The rhinoviruses are stable at pH 6–8; they are more sensitive to acid than the enteroviruses and cardioviruses, but less than foot and mouth disease virus. (Medappa *et al.,* 1971; Stott and Killington, 1973.)

RIF (resistance-inducing factors) (transformation-defective avian leukosis viruses).

Rift Valley fever virus (unclassified arbovirus). 60–90 nm spheres, ether sensitive, density 1.23 g/ml (disease of sheep, goats, and cattle).

Rinderpest virus (bovine paramyxovirus). Closely related to canine distemper and human measles virus. The two animal viruses are serologically related. Rinderpest virus contains a helical nucleocapsid similar to all members of this group.

RNA tumor viruses, *see* oncornavirus group.

Ross River virus (alphavirus subgroup of togaviridiae).

Rous sarcoma virus (avian oncornavirus). 80–120 nm particles (500–600 S) consisting of a dense nucleoprotein core (40 nm diameter) and a lipid-containing envelope with knoblike projections. The composition of the virion is 64% protein, 1.9% RNA, 1–2% carbohydrate; the rest is mostly lipid. The virus spectrum in 0.2% SDS, added to abolish the strong light scattering, shows a shallow maximum at 270 nm (260/280 absorbance ratio 1.15) A_{270} (0.1%) is about 2.0.

The phospholipid (31%) consists of sphingomyelin, phosphatidylcholine, and phosphatidylethanolamine, 1:1:1, similar but not identical to the phospholipid distribution in plasma membrane of infected and noninfected host (CEF) cells and of envelopes of Sindbis virus, Sendai virus, and Newcastle disease virus grown on the same cells. Thus the lipids are largely derived from, and determined by, the host.

The RNA (about 0.5% and containing about 2.5% poly(A)) is 60–70 S, corresponding to about 12×10^6 daltons per particle. Smaller RNA material also occurs in the virus (12–4 S, containing degradation products as well as 7 S, 5 S, and 4 S species). Upon melting (heat, dimethylsulfoxide, etc.) the large component becomes largely 35–30 S, believed to be due to release of unique molecules of RNA of 3–4 × 10^6 dalton molecular weight, held together by complementary H-bonded segments. A slightly larger and a smaller RNA component (a and b) have been found associated with nondefective viruses (producing foci in chick embryo fibroblasts) and avian leukosis viruses, respectively. The main proteins are two glycoproteins (105,000 and 36,000) in the envelope, probably making up the external spikes and carrying the type-specific antigens, and in the 50 nm diameter core proteins of 27,000, 19,000, 15,000, and 12,000 mol. wt., components of the group-specific antigen.

The glycoproteins differ slightly in size in a manner correlating with the presence of RNA components a and b. The glycopeptides obtained by exhaustive pronase treatment are of about 5700 and 3900 daltons, respectively.

The inner filamentous nucleoid liberated by Nonidet P40 (130 S, density in CsCl 1.34 g/ml) consists of only five of the eleven proteins detected in this study, the 28,000 protein predominating, and 20% RNA (30 4 S RNA molecules per 10^7 daltons of large-molecular-weight RNA). The nucleoid covered by an internal membrane represents the core of the virus.

Proteins associated with this membrane and the envelope are said to have molecular weights of 115 and 37 × 10^3, the smaller ones present in greatest numbers (2000–6000 per particle). Only the 14,000 mol. wt. protein appears strictly associated with the RNA. The reverse transcriptase of the virus (Prague strain), less than 2% of the soluble proteins of the virus and not containing carbohydrate, was of 6 S (after RNase treatment), probably 110,000 in molecular weight.

RSV and other virulent RNA tumor viruses are produced and excreted by the cells they transform. (Bolognesi *et al.*, 1972; Lai and Duesberg, 1972; Hung *et al.*, 1971.)

RPL-12 virus (transformation-defective avian leukosis virus) (Davis and Rueckert, 1972.)

RT virus (parvovirus).

Rubella virus (alphavirus subgroup of togaviridiae). Causes German measles in man, of particular danger during pregnancy. Only monkeys are susceptible. The pleomorphic enveloped lipid-containing 60 nm diameter particles contain a 150 S nucleocapsid with single-stranded RNA of about 3.4 × 10^6 daltons (39 S), of density 1.634 g/ml. Three proteins of 62,500, 48,000, and 35,000 daltons have been detected, the first two representing glycoproteins and the last the capsid protein. This pattern resembles that of the alphaviruses. The virus hemagglutinates at low temperatures only. The virus is not arthropod-transmitted. (Liebhaber and Gross, 1972; Vaheri and Hovi, 1972.)

Russian tick-borne (or spring-summer) encephalitis virus (flavivirus subgroup of togaviridiae). Related to louping ill virus.

R.V. (parvovirus). 3.6×10^6 dalton particles, containing 34% of single-stranded DNA (27 S) (1.3 [?] $\times 10^6$ mol. wt.).

SA 6 and SA 8 viruses (cercopithecid herpesvirus 2 and 3).

SA 7 virus (oncogenic simian adenovirus).

SA 11 virus, from South African *Cercopithecus* monkeys (orbivirus subgroup of reoviridiae). 72 nm enveloped particles. 57 nm in diameter when lacking outer shell, probably composed of 32 capsomeres. (Els and Lecatsas, 1972.)

Sacbrood virus (insect picornavirus similar but not related to bee acute paralysis viruses). Spherical particles, 28 nm in diameter (160 S). Contains 35% RNA (35 S), A/G/U/C = 32/19/31/18. Infects only bee larvae. (Newman *et al.,* 1973.)

Sacramento river chinook disease virus (rhabdovirus of salmon).

Salivary virus of bat (US) (flavivirus subgroup of togaviridiae).

San Miguel sea lion virus, probably identical with vesicular exanthema virus of swine.

Schmidt–Ruppin virus (nondefective avian sarcoma virus).

Scrapie agent of sheep, member of a group of not typical viruses, also called unconventional viruses (Kuru and Creutzfeld–Jakob disease of man and transmissible mink encephalopathy; possibly viroids). (Marx, 1973.)

Semliki Forest virus (alphavirus subgroup of togaviridiae). Spherical particles of 70–80 nm diameter (300–350 S), coated with a membrane and ether sensitive. Virus remains infectious after enzymatic removal of surface projections, but loses its hemagglutinating activity. The cores found in infected cells (40 nm diameter) (140 S) contain the RNA encapsidated in ribonuclease-resistant manner.

The RNA (6.3%) is 45 S and has a molecular weight of 4.1×10^6. Its composition is A/G/U/C = 29/26/20/25.

The single core protein (12%) has a molecular weight of 32,000, N-terminal lysine, and a high content of hydrophilic amino acids. The surface protein (44%, 2.5 moles/mole capsid protein) occurs as spikes exterior to the lipid envelope. It contains sugars (14%) and is of 54,000 mol. wt. with N-terminal valine. A part of the protein particularly rich in hydrophobic amino acids is anchored to the lipid envelope. The bilayered lipids in the envelope resemble those of the host cell plasma membrane, infected or uninfected, but with much less fatty acids and more cholesterol (0.41 mg lipid/mg protein, 31% neutral, 61% phospholipid, 8% glycolipid). (Acheson and Tamm, 1970.)

Sendai virus or hemagglutinating virus of Japan (parainfluenza subgroup of paramyxoviruses). Infects swine, mouse, and man. 150 nm diameter particles containing a 1100-nm-long helical nucleocapsid (5.0 nm pitch, about twelve protein subunits/turn) (see Electron micrograph VIII). The RNA is 50 S, about 6×10^6 in molecular weight, and 6.5 μm long. (A report that it can be dissociated into smaller components has been corrected.) It contains poly(A). Its composition is A/G/U/C = 24/23/30/23. (Kolakofsky *et al.*, 1974.)

Two glycoproteins containing fucose, galactose, and glucosamine are 65 and 53×10^3 daltons. The main capsid protein is 60×10^3 daltons, and a membrane protein is 38×10^3 daltons. Three additional proteins are of 72, 57, and 46×10^3 daltons. Sendai virus, like all paramyxoviruses, causes at high-multiplicity rapid formation of polykaryons by fusion of cell membranes. Trypsin is said to release "monovalent" hemagglutinin and fully active neuraminidase of 124×10^3 daltons and 114×10^3 daltons, apparently dimers of the above-listed glycoproteins. The neuraminidase of Sendai virus shows considerable similarity, in enzymatic and serological respects, to that of Newcastle disease virus (Iida, 1972; Mountcastle *et al.*, 1971.)

Sericestis iridescent virus (insect iridovirus, related to tipula iridescent virus). Icosahedral particles with 86-nm-long edges; diameter about 130 nm; 760×10^6 particle weight; consisting of probably 1562 protein subunits in outer shell. Contains double-stranded DNA (18%) of 134×10^6 mol. wt. (Glitz *et al.*, 1968.)

Sheep enterovirus (picornavirus). 28 nm diameter particle.

Sheeppox virus (subgroup of poxviruses).

Sheep pulmonary adenomatosis virus (herpesvirus). Also termed Jaagsiekte virus.

Shipping fever virus, *see* parainfluenza viruses.

Shope fibroma virus, *see* rabbit fibroma virus.

Shope (rabbit) papilloma virus (prototype for papilloma virus subgroup of papovaviridiae). Icosahedral particles of 53 nm diameter, about 50×10^6 particle weight. The architecture of the particle is probably the same as for polyoma virus: 72 capsomeres, $T = 7$; left-handed skew configuration. The sedimentation rates of the nucleocapsids and the empty capsids are 298 S and 172 S, respectively. The capsomeres are short (10 nm) hollow cylinders composed of five or six subunits. Double-stranded cyclic DNA of 5×10^6 mol. wt. and 48% (G+C). *See* under papilloma virus for more detailed information. (Klug and Finch, 1968.)

Sigma virus (rhabdovirus of *Drosophila*). 160×70 nm bullet-shaped particles.

Simian hemorrhagic fever virus (flavivirus subgroup of togaviridiae). Unrelated to other known viruses. 40–45 nm particles.

Simian herpesviruses (several of them, e.g., type 8, deadly also to man), *see* herpesvirus ateles, saimiri, simiae, tamarinus.

Simian paramyxoviruses, *see* SV-5, SV-41.

Simian sarcoma virus type 1 (oncornavirus). Typical C-type particles containing RNA of 60–70 S, 28 S, 18 S, and 4 S, and reverse transcriptase.

Simian viruses, *see* under SV.

Simian virus SA-11, *see* SA-11 virus.

Sindbis virus (alphavirus subgroup of togaviridiae, related to western equine encephalitis virus). Slightly pathogenic in man; transmitted by mosquitos. The 70 nm diameter particle contains a 40 nm core composed of 32 hexamer–pentamer morphological units ($T = 3$). The virus sediments with 273 S, the core with 173 S (see Electron micrograph XII).

The single-stranded RNA represents according to some authors a single chain without breaks of 42 S and a molecular weight of 4.3 $\times$ 10^6 daltons. Others are equally insistent that this is the dimer of a 26–28 S RNA, although it now appears probable that the latter is the sedimentation rate of the messenger RNA, the complementary form to the virion RNA (or part thereof). The composition of the viral RNA is A/G/U/C = 30/26/20/25. Sindbis RNA also contains poly(A) sequences of various lengths.

The viral envelope was recently shown to consist of two rather than one glycolipoproteins. The lipid and to a lesser extent the carbohydrate compositions vary depending on host and culture conditions (like those of myxo-, paramyxo-, and oncornaviruses). Both glycolipoproteins are of approximately 53,000 mol. wt., the capsid protein 30,000. All proteins arise by posttranslational cleavage from a large precursor protein. (Boulton and Westaway, 1972; Schlesinger and Schlesinger, 1972.)

Slow viruses, a not well defined group of viruses which are intermittently or continuously present in appreciable quantities in the infected host, and may but need not cause diseases of usually very chronic and degenerative nature, often associated with the central nervous system. Some human diseases have been attributed to slow viruses. They are probably related to oncornaviruses since they contain reverse transcriptases. *See* Visna virus, Maedi virus, lactic dehydrogenase virus, possibly Creutzfeld–Jakob, Kuru, etc.

Spidermonkey herpesvirus, cebid herpesvirus 3

Spondweni virus (flavivirus subgroup of togaviridiae).

Spring viremia virus of carp (rhabdovirus). Buoyant density in sucrose 1.16 g/ml. Contains 3 main proteins of 70, 40, and 19 $\times$ 10^3 daltons (9:4:4) and a small amount of a 150 $\times$ 10^3 species. Whether this agent causing infectious dropsy and the agent causing swim bladder inflammation are the same or closely related is as yet uncertain. (Bachmann and Ahne, 1973, Lenoir, 1973.)

Squirrel fibroma virus (myxoma subgroup of poxviruses).

St. Louis encephalitis virus (flavivirus subgroup of togaviridiae). The RNA is said to be of 3.3 $\times$ 10^6 daltons. A/G/U/C = 31/26/21/22. The BHK strain contains three proteins: 63,000 and 8500 mol. wt. in the envelope and 18,000 for the capsid protein; the Vero and BS strains contain proteins of 52,000 and 14,000 respectively. (Qureshi and Trent, 1972.)

Stratford virus (flavivirus subgroup of togaviridiae).

Subacute sclerosing panencephalitis virus (slow virus?, or para-myxovirus related to measles virus). However, papovavirus-like particles have also been found associated with this disease. Attacks central nervous system of children. Free nucleocapsids in infected tissue (both nucleus and cytoplasm) characterize this infection. They occur both in a helical form (18 nm diameter, 5–6 nm pitch, and 1.0 to 1.4 μm long) containing 4.3% RNA (density in CsCl 1.31 g/ml) and as granular 22–25 μm filaments. (Yeh and Iwasaki, 1972.)

SV-1 (oncogenic simian adenovirus).

SV-5 (simian parainfluenza subgroup of paramyxoviruses). The virus consists of 73% protein, 20% lipid, 6% carbohydrate, and 0.9% RNA. Its main protein components are a capsid and a membrane protein (61 and 41 $\times$ 10^3 daltons), and two glycoproteins (67 and 56 $\times$ 10^3) containing glucose, galactose, mannose, fucose, and glucosamine. Both neuraminidase and hemagglutinin activity were found associated with the larger of these two proteins (8.9 S). The glycolipid contains glucose, galactosamine, and galactose and lacks neuraminic acid. (Scheid *et al.*, 1972.)

SV-12 from monkeys, identical with human reovirus type 1.

SV-15 (nononcogenic simian adenovirus).

SV-20, 23, 25, 33, 34, 37, 38 (oncogenic simian adenoviruses).

SV-40 (simian polyoma virus). Particle dimensions and architecture as in polyoma virus (see Electron micrograph IX). The virus contains 12% double-stranded circular DNA of 3.2 $\times$ 10^6 mol. wt. (partly supercoiled), 41% (G+C), and one or possibly two capsid proteins of about 44 $\times$ 10^3 mol. wt. (75%), and two smaller proteins (32 and 23 $\times$ 10^3, 9 and 10%), as well as lesser amounts of yet smaller proteins (some possibly cellular histones) of 14,000, 12,500, and 11,000, 6000, and 4000 mol. wt. The virus contains an endonuclease which causes nicks in the DNA. All the major proteins are said to be phosphoproteins. (See Table 1 for amino acid analyses.)

SV-40 is lytic in monkey cells, and temperate, causing occasional transformation, in mouse cells. The isolated DNA is able to infect and to transform susceptible cells. Evidence has been presented that the agent causing progressive multifocal leukoencephalopathy (PML-2) in man is a variant of SV-40. (Tan and Sokol, 1972.)

SV-41 (simian parainfluenza subgroup of paramyxoviruses). Very similar to SV-5.

SV-59 from monkeys, identical with human reovirus type 2.

Swim bladder inflammation agent of carp (rhabdovirus). (Bachmann and Ahne, 1973.)

Swinefever virus (flavivirus subgroup of togaviridiae). Isometric virions of 40 nm diameter with a 29 nm core, 108 S, and of 1.17 g/ml density in CsCl. Contains RNA.

Swine influenza virus (myxovirus).

Swinepox virus (unclassified poxvirus).

Syncytium-forming ("foamy") type 3 virus (member of slow virus group resembling oncornaviruses). Simian, feline, etc., types have been observed. The virus contains reverse transcriptase and causes extensive cell fusion. (*See* "foamy" virus.)

Takaribe, Tamiani viruses (arenaviruses).

Tanapox virus of primates, similar to Yaba virus.

Termite paralysis virus (picornavirus).

Theilen feline sarcoma virus, *see* feline leukemia sarcoma virus.

Tick-borne encephalitis virus (Central European and Far Eastern subgroups; flavivirus subgroup of togaviridiae). Affects man.

Tipula iridescent virus (prototype of iridovirus of insects). Icosahedral particles of 130 nm diameter (2200 S), 82 nm edge length, probably containing 1472 protein subunits in outer coat (see Electron micrograph V). Double-stranded DNA of 126×10^6 mol. wt. (15%). Contains several proteins, little (9%) or no lipid. (Glitz *et al.,* 1968.)

TOGAVIRIDIAE. Family of very many viruses including most formerly called arboviruses. Subgroups, roughly corresponding to the A and B groups of the arboviruses, are the slightly larger (40–80 nm diameter) alphaviruses and the slightly smaller (30–50 nm diameter) flaviviruses.

The togaviruses are medium sized (usually 50–70 nm) enveloped viruses containing single-stranded RNA (see Electron micrograph XII). The RNAs of the togaviruses serve directly as messengers and appear to contain 3′-terminal polyadenylic acid sequences and no polymerases or transcriptases (RNA or DNA or reverse). The viruses mature by budding through the plasma membrane. They hemagglutinate red cells. The nonhemagglutinating nucleocapsids of 40 nm diameter are probably icosahedral, with 32 capsomeres. The protein composition of the togaviridiae is generally simple (about three, including the lipid-rich envelope proteins). (*See* rubella, Sindbis, Semliki Forest virus, etc.).

Toluca 1 virus (enterovirus). Serologically distinct from other known enteroviruses. Particles of 25 nm diameter.

Transmissible gastroenteritis virus of pigs (coronavirus).

Transmissible mink encephalopathy agent, *see* scrapie.

Tribec virus (orbivirus subgroup of reoviridiae).

Turkey herpesvirus 1, used to vaccinate against Marek's disease.

Turkeypox virus (birdpox subgroup of poxviruses).

TVX virus (parvovirus). Same properties as, though serologically differentiable from, KBSH virus.

Uganda S virus (flavivirus subgroup of togaviridiae).

Una virus (alphavirus subgroup of togaviridiae).

US bat salivary virus (flavivirus subgroup of togaviridiae).

Usutu virus (flavivirus subgroup of togaviridiae).

Uukuniemi virus (togavirus, separate serological group). 450 S particles, density 1.20 g/ml; contains RNA of 18 S, 21 S, and 27 S (4.1, 1.9, 0.9, and 0.8×10^6 daltons), and at least one envelope protein (70,000 mol. wt.) forming 8-nm-long projections, and one capsid protein (25,000 mol. wt.), seemingly forming a helix upon release, with a 9 nm diameter. The phospholipid content of the envelope is very similar to that of Semliki Forest virus grown on the same cells. (Pettersson *et al.*, 1971.)

Vaccinia virus of man (vaccinia subgroup of poxviruses). The approximately 200×300 nm particles ($\sim 6000 \times 10^6$ daltons) of complex structure are composed of 92% protein, 3% DNA, 5% lipid (cholesterol 1.2, phospholipid 2.1, neutral fat 1.7%), and 0.2% nondeoxyribose carbohydrate (in glycoproteins) (see Electron micrograph X). The double-stranded DNA is of $160–200 \times 10^6$ mol. wt. and 36% (G+C). 31 proteins have been seen (mol. wt. 130,000–8000): 5 near surface; 17 including two main protein components in cores which make up half of the virion; 2 glycoproteins of uncertain location; 6 phosphoproteins. The cores contain an RNA polymerase which transcribes 15% of the genome. One of the phosphoproteins of molecular weight 11,000 is associated with the core. (Sarov and Joklik, 1972.)

Vacuolating virus (or agent) (polyoma virus). Simian and rabbit forms are known; *see* SV-40.

Varicella-zoster virus (human herpesvirus 3). The virus causes both chickenpox and herpes zoster. The particle is of 200 nm diameter, 100 nm when not enveloped, and contains a dense core. The DNA has a density of 1.705 g/ml (compared to 1.717 for herpes simplex virus and 1.697 for host cellular DNA). (Gershon *et al.*, 1973; Taylor-Robinson and Caunt, 1972.)

Variola (minor) virus, smallpox virus (vaccinia subgroup of poxviruses). Possibly identical with alastrim virus.

Venezuelan equine encephalitis virus (alphavirus subgroup of togaviridiae). 60–75 nm particles with a 30–40 nm core. The phospholipid varies with and partially reflects that of the host's plasma membrane. There are considerable similarities among the lipids of different togaviruses. The lipids contribute to the relative heat resistance of these viruses. The RNA is of 40 S, 4.2×10^6 in molecular weight, and has a buoyant density in CsCl of 1.66 g/ml. (Heydrick *et al.*, 1971.)

Vesicular exanthema virus of swine (calicivirus subgroup of picornaviridiae). Isometric 35–40 nm diameter particles, 207 S, of density 1.38 g/ml. Contains 20% single-stranded RNA ($2–3 \times 10^6$ mol. wt.; 37 S) and 80% protein. A/G/U/C = 29/21/25/25. Virus is ether resistant, sensitive to acid (pH 3), and heat (50°C); not inhibited by actinomycin D. (Oglesby *et al.*, 1971.)

Vesicular stomatitis virus of cattle (prototype of rhabdovirus group). Bullet-shaped enveloped particles of 290×75 nm (625 S). The buoyant density in CsCl is 1.18 g/ml, the particle weight 385×10^6 daltons. Indiana serotype: 64% protein, 13% carbohydrate, 20% lipid, 3% RNA (see Electron micrograph XI). The RNA of about 45 S and molecular weight 4.2×10^6 has the composition A/G/U/C = 27/21/31/22. The RNA is single-stranded.

    The lipid composition, high particularly in phosphatidylethanolamine and sphingomyelin, is similar to that of other viral lipids (paramyxo-, myxo-, and togaviruses), and resembles the composition of the host cell plasma membrane more (but not entirely) than that of the entire host cell.

The glycolipid composition is similar to that of the host cell plasma membrane (neuraminic acid, galactose, glucose, ceramide) and represents host cell antigens. Most of the neuraminic acid is in the glycoprotein (G protein of about 69,000 daltons) making up the 10-nm-long spikes which is the major antigenic determinant of the intact virion, while the M protein (29,000–34,000 daltons) is situated in the underlying membrane.

The nucleocapsid is of 140 S, 3.5 nm long, and consists of 1000 protein subunits (density 1.32 g/ml). It contains 43 S single-stranded RNA of 4×10^6 mol. wt., which represents the "negative" strand and is thus noninfective when isolated. The RNA is transcribed by a virion RNA polymerase. The main protein of the nucleocapsid is the N protein (50,000–60,000 daltons). The largest protein (L, about 190,000 daltons) appears to represent the transcriptase, which does not also serve as replicase. The role of a "nonstructural" internal protein (NS, 40,000–45,000 daltons) is not clear; only the latter is a phosphoprotein. The virion also contains a protein kinase.

A comparative study of the two main serotypes (Indiana and New Jersey) as well as the Cocal virus indicates small differences between them. The molecular weight of the three major and one minor proteins are given in that study as about 62,000, 46,000, 27,000, and 38,000. Cocal is related more closely to the Indiana serotype.

The vesicular stomatitis virus replicates in mammals and arthropods. (Wagner *et al.*, 1972.)

Viral hemorrhagic septicemia virus (rhabdovirus of trout).

Visna virus of sheep (a member of slow virus group). A neurotropic variant of Maedi virus. The single-stranded RNA is about 63 S and 4 S, the former becoming about 35 S upon melting. The virus contains reverse transcriptase and DNA-dependent DNA polymerase activities. It transforms murine cells. Among its 11–14 proteins (mol. wt. 142,000–14,000) are at least 2 glycoproteins, the pattern resembling that of the oncornavirus proteins. (Mountcastle *et al.*, 1972.)

von Magnus virus (defective form of influenza virus), *see* defective virus.

Wad Medani, Wallal, and Warrego viruses (orbivirus subgroup of reoviridiae).

Wart virus, *see* human papilloma virus.

Wesselsbron virus (flavivirus subgroup of togaviridiae). Affects sheep.

Western equine encephalitis virus (alphavirus subgroup of togaviridiae). A/G/U/C = 30/22/23/25.

West Nile virus (flavivirus subgroup of togaviridiae).

Whataroa virus (alphavirus subgroup of togaviridiae). Related to Western equine encephalitis virus.

Woolly monkey sarcoma virus (oncornavirus).

X-14 virus (parvovirus).

Yaba virus of monkey (poxvirus). Double-stranded DNA has density of 1.6905, 32.5% (G+C). Oncogenic. Contains several enzymes. (Schwartz and Dales, 1971.)

Yellow fever virus (flavivirus subgroup of togaviridiae).

Yucaipa virus (paramyxovirus). Symptoms range from inapparent disease to death. Contains neuraminidase.

Zika virus (flavivirus subgroup of togaviridiae).

TABLE 1

Amino Acid Composition of Animal Virus Coat Proteins (Pure Single Chain Components)*

	Asp	Thr	Ser	Glu	Pro	Gly	Ala	Cys	Val	Met	Ile	Leu	Tyr	Phe	Lys	His	Arg	Trp
Picornaviruses																		
EMC 1 (=α?)	8.9	7.0	13.0	10.7	5.3	15.1	6.7	ND	5.4	ND	3.1	6.3	1.7	4.4	4.9	3.0	4.4	ND
EMC 2 (=β?)	10.1	10.0	10.0	9.5	8.8	10.5	7.3	ND	8.1	ND	3.6	8.1	3.4	8.1	5.2	2.1	4.1	ND
EMC 4 (=γ?)	8.6	9.6	8.7	9.0	7.1	9.8	8.4	ND	7.0	ND	4.2	7.0	3.2	5.4	4.5	2.4	4.1	ND
ME α	9.2	7.7	9.9	9.7	7.0	10.7	6.0	1.6	6.9	0.9	2.9	6.9	2.8	5.6	4.7	1.8	3.7	ND
ME β	10.1	9.7	8.1	10.1	5.1	8.9	7.7	0.7	6.9	1.5	3.5	7.8	2.9	3.9	3.5	2.9	4.8	ND
ME γ	7.5	10.1	10.1	7.1	8.3	9.2	8.8	1.2	5.5	2.1	5.2	6.7	4.2	4.4	4.0	1.1	2.9	1.6
ME δ	19.6	4.2	16.6	8.5	4.3	9.0	7.6	0	2.9	1.0	3.7	8.7	3.1	4.2	2.2	0.3	2.0	ND
Influenza virus																		
Neuraminidase																		
Lee strain (type B)	10.0	8.2	7.6	7.9	4.7	9.6	6.6	2.7	5.0	2.5	5.6	8.8	3.9	2.8	6.8	2.6	4.8	ND
Bel strain (type A$_0$)	11.9	6.1	9.5	10.5	4.7	9.4	4.5	2.4	6.7	0.9	8.6	6.3	2.5	3.9	6.3	1.8	3.9	ND
X-7F$_1$	14.5	7.1	10.3	8.7	4.9	9.1	3.8	2.6	7.3	1.1	8.5	4.7	2.4	3.3	4.5	1.2	6.1	ND
A2,1957†	13.7	5.7	10.9	7.4	4.3	9.5	2.8	3.9	6.7	1.7	6.3	3.5	2.3	2.8	3.7	1.9	5.6	none
Hemagglutinin																		
Lee strain, heavy chain	11.4	8.6	6.1	8.4	7.0	10.1	4.4	1.8	6.8	0.8	6.7	7.3	2.9	2.3	8.7	2.4	4.3	ND
Lee strain, light chain	13.1	5.6	7.6	9.7	1.8	9.0	9.4	1.2	4.2	1.1	6.5	13.6	1.3	3.2	6.2	3.5	3.1	ND
Bel strain, heavy chain	11.7	7.2	9.2	11.3	4.6	8.5	5.5	1.5	6.0	0.5	6.6	8.9	3.4	3.3	5.8	2.0	4.8	ND
Bel strain, light chain	13.9	4.5	7.8	13.3	0.5	10.6	5.6	1.1	6.0	0.8	6.0	9.6	3.6	4.3	8.0	1.6	2.7	ND

Capsid																		
Lee strain	12.0	6.0	7.3	9.9	3.4	8.9	8.3	0.0	5.2	1.9	7.5	9.6	1.8	3.5	8.8	0.9	5.1	ND
Bel strain	8.6	5.6	6.8	15.2	3.9	8.2	8.0	0.8	5.4	1.4	6.3	8.7	1.7	4.3	5.7	1.3	8.3	ND
Lee strain M‡	8.2	3.8	6.6	12.2	1.8	8.8	9.0	1.4	4.8	3.8	5.2	12.0	2.0	3.1	9.5	2.1	5.6	ND
Bel strain M‡	7.5	6.5	5.8	16.2	3.4	6.6	10.3	0.5	6.4	2.0	4.8	12.0	1.0	2.6	5.6	1.8	7.2	ND
Reovirus																		
λ1 + λ2	12	7.4	7.9	9.4	5.4	6.2	7.8	ND	7.1	3.4	6.0	9.3	4.1	4.2	2.8	1.7	5.3	ND
μ2	9.5	7.2	8.8	9.9	6.9	6.2	9.6	0.7	7.3	2.4	5.6	7.8	2.9	2.5	5.4	0.7	3.8	2.4
σ2	10.7	7.2	8.0	10.7	4.3	8.3	9.5	ND	6.0	2.0	4.0	10.7	3.7	5.2	1.4	1.7	6.6	ND
σ3	12.0	4.7	6.6	9.1	5.4	8.2	6.0	0.6	8.5	2.8	3.5	8.5	2.8	3.5	5.0	3.7	5.7	3.2
Adenovirus																		
Hexon	15	7.2	6.9	11	6.1	7.2	7.9	0	5.5	2.1	3.6	7.6	5.9	4.9	4.0	1.1	4.2	ND
Fiber	10	8.8	8.8	5.0	4.4	6.9	5.0	0.6	4.4	1.2	3.8	7.5	2.5	2.5	5.0	0.6	1.2	1.2
Major core protein (mol. wt. 18,000)	6.8	7.3	4.2	4.8	6.7	7.8	20	10	4.4	0.6	2.4	3.4	0.4	0.4	2.9	0.5	23	ND
Celo hexon	17	8.0	6.2	8.5	6.1	7.5	6.6	0	7.4	1.4	3.6	8.3	4.7	5.1	2.9	1.4	5.2	ND
SV-40 *strain 777*																		
mol. wt.																		
VP 1 ~ 43,000	10.6	7.6	5.7	11.5	6.5	9.7	6.4	0?	9.2	1.8	4.1	9.1	2.6	3.7	6.5	1.6	3.6	ND
VP 3 ~ 26,000	7.9	4.2	7.1	11.5	5.2	18.2	6.6	0?	6.9	1.9	3.2	8.6	3.1	3.2	5.2	1.4	5.7	ND
VP 4 ~ 16,000	7.5	5.7	7.2	9.8	4.7	13.5	9.6	0?	6.9	2.5	5.0	8.7	2.8	3.2	7.5	0.8	5.8	ND
VP 5 ~ 13,000	7.2	5.3	7.1	8.0	3.6	15.7	10.7	0?	6.8	1.1	4.4	7.5	2.0	3.1	8.9	0.8	8.0	ND
VP 6 ~ 11,000	7.9	5.3	7.1	9.5	4.1	16.2	8.2	0?	7.6	2.0	4.5	8.1	3.2	4.0	6.6	0.8	5.2	ND

* All given as mole-percentages. To obtain approximate residues/mole data each figure has to be multiplied by the protein molecular weight/11,500. ND means not determined.

† Glucosamine 1.1; no galactosamine nor tryptophan detected.

‡ Membrane protein.

References (Section A)

Acheson, N. H., and Tamm, I., 1970, *Virology* **41**, 306, 321.

Almeida, J. D., Waterson, A. P., and Plowright, W., 1967, *Arch. ges. Virusforsch.* **20**, 392.

Andrewes, C., and Pereira, H. G., 1972, *Viruses of Vertebrates,* 3rd edition, Williams and Wilkins Co., Baltimore.

Appel, M. J. G., and Gillespie, J. H., 1972, *Canine Distemper Virus,* Virology Monographs No. 11, Springer-Verlag, New York.

Aubertin, A., Palese, P., Tan, K. B., Vilagines, R., and McAuslan, B. R., 1971, *J. Virol.* **8**, 643.

Bachmann, P. A., and Ahne, W., 1973, *Nature* **244**, 235.

Bachrach, H. L., Swaney, J. B., and vande Woude, G. F., 1973, *Virology* **52**, 520.

Bergoin, M., Devauchelle, G., and Vago, C., 1971, *Virology* **43**, 453.

Berns, K. I., and Adler, S., 1972, *J. Virol.* **9**, 394.

Bolognesi, D. P., Bauer, H., Gelderblom, H., and Hüper, G., 1972, *Virology* **47**, 551.

Borden, E. C., Shope, R. E., and Murphy, F. A., 1971, *J. Gen. Virol.* **13**, 261.

Boulton, R. W., and Westaway, E. G., 1972, *Virology* **49**, 283.

Brown, F., and Hull, R., 1973, *J. Gen. Virol.* **20** (suppl.), 43.

Burlingham, B. T., and Doerfler, W., 1972, *Virology* **48**, 1.

Butterworth, B. E., and Rueckert, R. R., 1972, *Virology* **50**, 535.

Carter, M. F., Biswal, N., and Rawls, W. E., 1973, *J. Virol.* **11**, 61.

Chen, J. H., Lee, L. F., Nazerian, K., and Burmester, B. R., 1972, *Virology* **47**, 434.

Clark, H. F., Michalski, F., Tweedell, K. S., Yohn, D., and Zeigel, R. F., 1973, *Virology* **51**, 392.

Clarke, J. K., and McFerran, J. B., 1971, *J. Gen. Virol.* **13**, 339.

Cunningham, C. H., Spring, M. P., and Nazerian, K., 1972, *J. Gen. Virol.* **16**, 423.

Darnell, M. B., and Plagemann, P. G. W., 1972, *J. Virol.* **10**, 1082.

Davis, N. L., and Rueckert, R. R., 1972, *J. Virol.* **10**, 1010.

Dreesman, G. R., Hollinger, F. B., Suriano, J. R., Fujioka, R. S., Brunschwig, J. P., and Melnick, J. L., 1972a, *J. Virol.* **10**, 469.

Dreesman, G. R., Suriano, J. R., Swartz, S. K., and McCombs, R. M., 1972b, *Virology* **50**, 528.

East, J. L., and Kingsbury, D. W., 1972, *J. Virol.* **8**, 161.

Eggen, K. L., and Shatkin, A. J., 1972, *J. Virol.* **9**, 636.

Els, H. J., and Lecatsas, G., 1972, *J. Gen. Virol.* **17**, 129.

Feinstone, S. M., Kapikian, A. Z., and Purceli, R. H., 1973, *Science* **182**, 1026.

Friedmann, T., and David, D., 1972, *J. Virol.* **10**, 776.

Fuscaldo, A. A., Aaslestad, H. G., and Hoffman, E. J., 1971, *J. Virol.* **7**, 233.

Gershon, A., Cosio, L., and Brunell, P. A., 1973, *J. Gen. Virol.* **18,** 21.

Gibson, W., and Roizman, B., 1972, *J. Virol.* **10,** 1044.

Gilden, R. V., Lee, Y. K., Oroszlan, S., Walker, J. L., and Huebner, R. J., 1970, *Virology* **41,** 187.

Glitz, D. G., Hills, G. J., and Rivers, C. F., 1968, *J. Gen. Virol.* **3,** 209.

Graham, B. J., Ludwig, H., Bronson, D. L., Benyesh-Melnick, M., and Biswal, N., 1972, *Biochem. Biophys. Acta* **259,** 13.

Granoff, A., 1972, *Fed. Proc.* **31,** 1626.

Györgi, E., Sheehan, M. C., and Sokol, F., 1971, *J. Virol.* **8,** 649.

Hall, W. W., and Martin, S. J., 1973, *J. Gen. Virol.* **19,** 175.

Harrap, K. A., 1972, *Virology* **50,** 114, 124.

Hess, W. R., 1971, *African Swine Fever,* Virology Monographs, Springer-Verlag, New York.

Hess, W., and Dardidi, A. H., 1968, *Arch. ges. Virusforsch.* **24,** 148.

Heydrick, F. P., Comer, J. F., and Wachter, R. F., 1971, *J. Virol.* **7,** 642.

Hierholzer, J. C., Palmer, E. L., Whitfield, S. G., Kaye, H. S., and Dowdle, W. R., 1972, *Virology* **48,** 516.

Hinze, H. C., and Chipman, P. J., 1972, *Fed. Proc.* **31,** 1639.

Holmes, I. H., 1971, *Virology* **43,** 708.

Horzinek, M. C., 1973, *J. Gen. Virol.* **20** (suppl.), 87.

Huang, A. S., Greenawalt, J. W., and Wagner, R., 1966, *Virology* **30,** 161.

Huang, E. S., Chen, S. T., and Pagano, J. S., 1973, *J. Virol.* **12,** 1473.

Hung, P. P., Robinson, H. L., and Robinson, W. S., 1971, *Virology* **43,** 251.

Hyllseth, B., 1973, *Arch. ges. Virol.* **40,** 177.

Iida, T., 1972, *J. Gen. Virol.* **14,** 69.

Ito, Y., Tanaka, Y., Inaba, Y., and Omori, T., 1973a, *Arch. ges. Virusforsch.* **40,** 29.

Ito, Y., Tanaka, Y., Inaba, Y., and Omori, T., 1973b, *Arch. ges. Virusforsch.* **40,** 198.

Jacquemont, B., Grange, J., Gazzolo, L., and Richard, M. H., 1972, *J. Virol.* **9,** 836.

Johnson, F. B., and Hoggan, M. D., 1973, *Virology* **51,** 129.

Joklik, W. K., 1972, *Virology* **49,** 700.

Karabatsos, N., 1973, *Arch. ges. Virusforsch.* **40,** 222.

Kelly, D. C., and Robertson, J. S., 1973, *J. Gen. Virol.* **20** (suppl.), 17.

Kelly, R. K., and Loh, P. C., 1972, *J. Virol.* **10,** 824.

Kingsbury, D. W., Portner, A., and Darlington, R. W., 1970, *Virology* **42,** 857.

Kinkelin, P. de, Galimard, B., and Bootsma, R., 1973, *Nature* **241,** 465.

Klenk, H. -D., and Rott, R., 1973, *J. Virol.* **11,** 823.

Klenk, H. -D., Rott, R., and Becht, H., 1972, *Virology* **47,** 579.

Klug, A., and Finch, J. T., 1968, *J. Molec. Biol.* **31,** 1.

Kolakofsky, D., Boy de la Tour, E., and Delius, H., 1974, *J. Virol.* **13,** 261.

Kurstak, E., Vernon, J. P., and Brakier-Gingras, L., 1973, *Arch. ges. Virusforsch.* **40,** 274.

Lai, M. M. C., and Duesberg, P. H., 1972, *Virology* **50,** 359.

Laver, W. G., and Baker, N., 1972, *J. Gen. Virol.* **17,** 61.

Laver, W. G., Younghusband, H. B., and Wrigley, N. G., 1971, *Virology* **45,** 598.

Lee, J. F., Armstrong, R. L., and Mazerian, K., 1972, *Avian Dis.* **16,** 799.

Lenoir, G., 1973, *Biochem. Biophys. Res. Comm.* **51,** 895.

Lewandowski, L. J., and Traynor, B. L. 1972, *J. Virol.* **10,** 1053.

Liebhaber, H., and Gross, P. A., 1972, *Virology* **47,** 684.

Lin, F. H., and Thormar, H., 1972, *J. Virol.* **10,** 228.

Longworth, J. F., Payne, C. C., and Macleod, R., 1973, *J. Gen. Virol.* **18,** 119.

Lyons, M. J., and Heyduk, J., 1973, *Virology* **54,** 37.

Madeley, C. R., Allan, W. H., and Kendall, A. P., 1971, *J. Gen. Virol.* **12,** 69.

Mak, S., 1971, *J. Virol.* **7,** 426.

Maldonado, R. L., and Bose, H. R., 1972, *J. Virol.* **8,** 813.

Maldonado, R. L., and Bose, H. R., 1973, *J. Virol.* **11,** 741.

Malmquist, W. A., van der Maaten, M. J., and Boothe, A. D., 1969, *Cancer Res.* **29,** 188.

Manning, J. S., and Hackett, A. J., 1972, *J. Nat. Cancer Inst.* **48,** 417.

Martin, S. J., and Johnston, M. D., 1972, *J. Gen. Virol.* **16,** 115.

Martin, S. A., and Zweerink, H. J., 1972, *Virology* **50,** 495.

Matsumura, T., Stollar, V., and Schlesinger, R. W., 1971, *Virology* **46,** 344.

Marx, J. L., 1973, *Science* **181,** 44.

McLerran, C. J., and Arlinghaus, R. B., 1973, *Virology* **53,** 247.

Medappa, K. C., McLean, C., and Rueckert, R. R., 1971, *Virology* **44,** 259.

Meléndez, L. V., Hunt, R. D., Daniel, M. D., Fraser, C. E. O., Barahona, H. H., King, N. W., and García, F. G., 1971, *Fed. Proc.* **31,** 1643.

Miller, R. L., and Plagemann, P. G. W., 1972, *J. Gen. Virol.* **17,** 349.

Molomut, N., Padnos, M., Gross, L., and Satory, V., 1964, *Nature* **204,** 1003.

Moroni, C., 1972, *Virology* **47,** 1.

Moss, D. J., and Pope, J. H., 1972, *J. Gen. Virol.* **17,** 233.

Mountcastle, W. E., Compans, R. W., and Choppin, P. W., 1971, *J. Virol.* **7,** 47.

Murphy, F. A., and Fields, B. N., 1967, *Virology* **33,** 625.

Murphy, F. A., Shope, R. E., Metselaar, D., and Simpson, D. I. H., 1970a, *Virology* **40,** 288.

Murphy, F. A., Scherer, W. F., Harrison, A. K., Dunne, H. W., and Gary, G. E. Jr., 1970b, *Virology* **40,** 1008.

Murphy, F. A., Borden, E. C., Shope, R. E., and Harrison, A., 1971, *J. Gen. Virol.* **13,** 273.

Nakajima, H., Tanaka, S., and Ushimi, C., 1970, *Arch. ges. Virusforsch.* **31,** 273.

Newman, J. F. E., Brown, F., Bailey, L., and Gibbs, A. J., 1973, *J. Gen. Virol.* **19,** 405.

Nichols, J. L., Quade, K., and Luftig, R. B., 1973, *J. Virol.* **11,** 432.

Nonoyama, M., Watanabe, Y., and Graham, A. F., 1970, *J. Virol.* **6,** 226.

Nowinski, R. C., Sarkar, N. H., Old, L. J., Moore, D. H., Scheer, D. I., and Hilgers, J., 1971, *Virology* **46,** 21.

Oglesby, A. S., Schaffer, F. L., and Madin, S. H., 1971, *Virology* **44,** 329.

Pedersen, I. R., 1973, *J. Virol.* **11,** 416.

Pett, D. M., Vanaman, T. C., and Joklik, W. K., 1973, *Virology* **52,** 174.

Pettersson, R., Kääriäinen, L., von Bonsdorff, C.-H., and Oker-Blom, N., 1971, *Virology* **46,** 721.

Phillips, B. A., 1972, *The Morphogenesis of Poliovirus,* Current Topics in Microbiology and Immunology, No. 58, Springer-Verlag, New York.

Pirie, G. D., Bishop, P. M., Burke, D. C., and Postlethwaite, R., 1971, *J. Gen. Virol.* **13,** 311.

Prage, L., and Pettersson, U., 1971, *Virology* **45,** 364.

Prage, L., Höglund, S., and Phillipson, L., 1972, *Virology* **49,** 745.

Qureshi, A. A., and Trent, D. W., 1972, *J. Virol.* **9,** 565.

Roblin, R., Härle, E., and Dulbecco, R., 1971, *Virology* **45,** 555.

Rowe, W. P., Murphy, F. A., Bergold, G. H., Casals, J., Hotchin, J., Johnson, K. M., Lehmann-Grube, F., Mims, C. A., Traub, E., and Webb, P. A., 1970, *J. Virol.* **5**, 651.

Saikku, P., von Bonsdorff, C.-H., Brummer-Korvenkontio, M., and Vaheri, A., 1971, *J. Gen. Virol.* **13**, 335.

Salzman, L. A., White, W. L., and Kakefuda, T., 1971, *J. Virol.* **7**, 830.

Sarkar, N. H., Nowinski, R. C., and Moore, D. H., 1971, *Virology* **46**, 1.

Sarov, I., and Joklik, W. K., 1972, *Virology* **50**, 579.

Schäfer, W., Lange, J., Fischinger, P. J., Frank, H., Bolognesi, D. P., and Pister, L., 1972, *Virology* **47**, 210.

Scheid, A., and Choppin, P. W., 1973, *J. Virol.* **11**, 263.

Scheid, A., Caliguiri, L. A., Compans, R. W., and Choppin, P. W., 1972, *Virology* **50**, 640.

Schlesinger, R. W., 1969, *Adv. Virus Res.* **14**, 1.

Schlesinger, S., and Schlesinger, M. J., 1972, *J. Virol.* **10**, 925.

Schluederberg, A., 1971, *Biochem. Biophys. Res. Comm.* **42**, 1012.

Schulze, I. T., 1972, *Virology* **47**, 181.

Schwartz, J., and Dales, S., 1971, *Virology* **45**, 797.

Shapiro, D., Brandt, W. E., Cardiff, R. D., and Russell, P. K., 1971, *Virology* **44**, 108.

Shimotohno, K., and Miura, K., 1973, *Virology* **53**, 283.

Siegert, R., 1972, *Marburg Virus,* Virology Monographs No. 11, Springer-Verlag, New York.

Siegl, B., Hallaner, C., Novak, A., and Kronauer, G., 1971, *Arch. ges. Virusforsch.* **35**, 91.

Sokol, F., and Clark, H. F., 1973, *Virology* **52**, 246.

Stollar, V., 1969, *Virology* **39**, 426.

Stoltz, D. B., and Summers, M. D., 1972, *J. Virol.* **8**, 900.

Stoltzfus, C. M., and Rueckert, R., 1972, *J. Virol.* **10**, 347.

Stone, L. B., Takemoto, K. K., and Martin, M. A., 1972, *J. Virol.* **8**, 573.

Stott, E. J., and Killington, R. A., 1973, *J. Gen. Virol.* **18**, 65.

Stromberg, K., 1972, *J. Virol.* **9**, 684.

Sukeno, N., Shirachi, R., Shiraishi, H., and Ishida, N., 1972, *J. Virol.* **10**, 157.

Summers, M. D., and Anderson, D. L., 1972, *Virology* **50**, 459.

Tan, K. B., and McAuslan, B. R., 1971, *Virology* **45**, 200.

Tan, K. B., and Sokol, F., 1972, *J. Virol.* **10**, 985.

Tanaka, Y., Inaba, Y., Sato, K., Ito, H., Omori, T., and Matumoto, M., 1969, *Japan J. Microbiol.* **13**, 169.

Tanaka, Y., Inaba, Y., Ito, Y., Sato, K., Omori, T., and Matumoto, M., 1972, *Japan J. Microbiol.* **16**, 95.

Tannock, G. A., Gibbs, A. J., and Cooper, P. D., 1970, *Biochem. Biophys. Res. Comm.* **38**, 298.

Tattersall, P., 1972, *J. Virol.* **10**, 586.

Taylor-Robinson, D., and Caunt, A. E., 1972, *Varicella Virus,* Virology Monographs No. 12, Springer-Verlag, New York.

Teninges, D., and Plus, N., 1972, *J. Gen. Virol.* **16**, 103.

Tinsley, T. W., and Longworth, J. F., 1973, *J. Gen. Virol.* **20** (suppl.), 7.

Vaheri, A., and Hovi, T., 1972, *J. Virol.* **9**, 10.

vande Woude, G. F., and Bachrach, H. L., 1971, *J. Virol.* **7**, 250.

van Frank, R. M., Ellis, L. F., and Kleinschmidt, W. J., 1971, *J. Gen. Virol.* **12**, 33.

Verwoerd, D. W., Els, H. J., de Villiers, E.-M., and Huismans, H., 1972, *J. Virol.* **10,** 783.

von Magnus, P., 1954, *Adv. Virus Res.* **2,** 59.

Wagner, G. W., Paschke, J. D., Campbell, W. R., and Webb, S. R., 1973, *Virology* **52,** 72.

Wagner, R. R., Prevec, L., Brown, F., Summers, D. F., Sokol, F., and MacLeod, R., 1972, *J. Virol.* **10,** 1228.

Walker, D. L., Padgett, B. L., ZuRhein, G. M., and Albert, A. E., 1973, *Science* **181,** 674.

Welsh, R. M., O'Connell, C. M., and Pfau, C. J., 1972, *J. Gen. Virol.* **17,** 355.

Wolf, K., and Darlington, R. W., 1972, *J. Virol.* **8,** 525.

Wood, H. A., Bozarth, R. F., and Mislivec, P. B., 1971, *Virology* **44,** 592.

Yang, S. S., and Wivel, N. A., 1973, *J. Virol.* **11,** 287.

Yau, T., and Rouhandeh, H., 1973, *Biochem. Biophys. Acta* **299,** 210.

Yeh, J., and Iwasaki, Y., 1972, *J. Virol.* **10,** 1220.

Zwillenberg, L. O., and Wolf, K., 1968, *J. Virol.* **2,** 393.

Section B

Plant Viruses

All plant viruses, except when noted, contain single-stranded RNA and most of them could with justification be classified as picornaviruses, because of their great similarities in structure and replication to the picornaviruses of vertebrates and insects as well as the small RNA phages. In most instances, the most common host represents part of the name of the plant viruses. Only when this is not the case will hosts be specifically mentioned. More complete biological characterization of many plant viruses is found in the Commonwealth Mycological Institute and Association of Applied Biologists (CMI/AAB) Description of Viruses. Those for which such information sheets are presently available are indicated by an asterisk.

Abaca mosaic virus (serologically related to sugarcane mosaic virus).

Agropyron mosaic virus* (similar but only distantly if at all related to hordeum and wheat streak mosaic virus, structurally similar to potato virus Y group). Filamentous 15 × 717 nm particles (165 S).

Alfalfa mosaic virus* (AMV) (synonym: lucerne mosaic virus) (prototype of a small group of stubby bacilliform multiparticle viruses or coviruses).† Four (or five) different RNA-containing particles of 18 nm × 58, 48, 36, and 18 nm, and 99, 89, 73, and 68 S (see Electron micrograph XIII). Also RNA-free particles. The particle weights range from 7.3×10^6 to 3.7×10^6. A_{260} (0.1%) = 5.2, the 260/280 nm absorbance ratio 1.75. The virions are quite sensitive

---

† I will use the term covirus for the ever-increasing number of virus isolates where two or more different component particles, which may or may not be easily separable, are required for infectivity (see *Coviruses* for listing).

to high salt and to ribonuclease action, but not particularly sensitive to elevated temperatures.

The RNA content is 18%. The largest particle contains an RNA molecule of 1.6×10^6 daltons, the others proportionately less. For the strain termed S (Strasbourg) RNA molecular weights of 1.3, 1.0, 0.7, and 0.34×10^6 (24 S, 20 S, 17 S, 12 S) have been reported. The average composition is A/G/U/C = 27/23/30/20.

In strain 425 the three largest virion particles of 95 S, 82 S, and 73 S were found necessary to achieve infectivity (not the 68 S and the 53 S RNA-free so-called top component). In contrast, all four of the RNA components were required.

The single coat protein of strain 15/64 was reported to have molecular weight 29,000 (see Table 2 for amino acid composition). The N- and C-chain termini of strain 425, of molecular weight 24,800, are AcSer- and -Arg-His, respectively; those of strain 15/64 are AcSer- and -Arg. Eight other strain proteins including 15/64 showed that same lower molecular weight.

About 200 mg virus can be obtained from 1 liter sap using tobacco as host. There exist many strains of alfalfa mosaic virus. It has a wide host range, growing in most legumes. Local lesion hosts for testing are common bean (*Phaseolus vulgaris*) and cowpea (*Vigna sinensis*). These viruses are transmittable mechanically, as well as by aphids, in which they do not persist. (Bol and Van Vloten-Doting, 1973.)

American wheat striate mosaic virus, *see* wheat striate mosaic virus.

Andean potato latent virus (very distant serological relationship to turnip yellow mosaic virus group; more closely related to belladonna mottle virus). Isometric particle containing 37% RNA of 2.55×10^6 daltons; A/G/U/C = 22/15/29/34. (Bercks *et al.*, 1971.)

Annulus tabaci, synonym for tobacco ringspot virus.

Annulus zonatus, synonym for tomato ringspot virus.

Apple chlorotic leaf spot (or latent) virus* (similar but not serologically related to apple stem grooving virus). Filamentous particles of 12×600 nm, 96 S, helical pitch 3.8 nm. The 260/280 nm absorbance ratio is quite unusual for a virus containing about 5% RNA (said to be about 1.8). The virus is labile and ribonuclease sensitive. It is propagated and tested on *Chenopodium quinoa*. (Lister and Hadidi, 1971.)

Apple latent virus 2, synonym for sowbane mosaic virus.

Apple mosaic virus* (multiparticle picornavirus, similar but not serologically related to tobacco streak virus; serologically related to prunus necrotic ringspot virus). Two sizes of 25–30 nm labile nucleoprotein particles, 88 S and 117 S, as well as a nucleic-acid-free "top component" are observed. Only the largest particle is infective, but covirus relationship has not been ruled out. The 260/280 nm absorbance ratio is 1.50. The virus contains 16% RNA. (Fulton, 1967, 1968.)

Apple stem grooving virus* (similar but not serologically related to apple chlorotic leaf spot virus). Very flexuous particles, 14 × 619 nm, 112 S, of 3.8 nm helical pitch. The 260/280 absorbance ratio is 1.18. The isoelectric point is pH 4.3. The virus is quite stable. It is propagated and tested on *Chenopodium quinoa.* (de Sequeira and Lister, 1969.)

Apple (Tulare) mosaic virus,* *see* Tulare apple mosaic virus.

Arabis mosaic virus* (multiparticle picornavirus, distantly serologically related to grapevine fanleaf virus, structurally similar to tobacco ringspot virus group).

Typical icosahedral particles of about 30 nm diameter and two sedimentation rates: 93 S, containing 28% RNA and particle weight 5.6 × 10⁶; and 126 S, containing 41% RNA of 5.5 × 10⁶ particle weight. There is also an RNA-free "top component" (53 S). The protein has a molecular weight of 53,500.

The virus is transmitted mechanically and by nematode vectors. Infection is associated with characteristic inclusion bodies. (Agrawal, 1967.)

Artichoke curly dwarf virus (member of potato virus X group).

Artichoke mottle crinkle virus (member of tomato bushy stunt virus group).

Aster ringspot virus, strain of tobacco rattle virus.

Atropa mild mosaic virus (a strain or synonym of henbane mosaic virus). Slightly flexuous threads (rods), 14 × 925 nm. The virus is transmitted mechanically and by aphid vectors; in the main host, tobacco, it produces "pinwheel-like" inclusion bodies in the infected cell.

Aucuba mosaic viruses (yellow and green aucuba mosaic virus, closely related strains of tobacco mosaic virus). These viruses form characteristic inclusion bodies in infected cells which actually represent virus crystals of three different types. The coat proteins of the aucuba strains differ from that of wild type TMV in only a few (e.g., three) amino acid replacements.

Barley (false) stripe virus* (rod-shaped virus unrelated to other known rod-shaped viruses). Particles of 20×128 nm (185 S), also in part 110 and 148 nm long, with 2.5 nm helical pitch. Probably a multicomponent covirus. The predominant particle weight is 26×10^6; the isoelectric point pH 4.5 The virus contains 4% RNA of molecular weight 10^6 (21 S); $A/G/U/C = 31/20/29/19$.

$A_{max(=271)}$ (0.1%) = 2.7, the 260/280 nm absorbance ratio 1.03. This is the only plant virus with an absorbance maximum not at 260 nm. This is due to its containing only 4% RNA, and contrasts it to viruses with 5% RNA (e.g., TMV), which show a slight decrease in absorbance from 260 to 270 nm. The protein has a molecular weight of 21,500; it is a glycoprotein.

The virus is seed transmitted. It has a moderate host range among mono- and dicotyledons; it gives local lesions suitable for quantitation on *Chenopodium amaranticolor* and *C. album* (ornamental goosefoot and lamb's quarter), as well as on Samsun tobacco. (Atabekov *et al.*, 1968; Jackson and Brakke, 1973.)

Barley yellow dwarf virus* (similar and possibly related serologically to beet western yellows virus). At least three serotypes exist. Dense polyhedral 27 nm, 117 S particles; 260/280 nm absorbance ratio 1.92. Contains 2×10^6 dalton (33 S) RNA. This rather unstable virus and related strains are economically important; they are transmitted only by aphids, in which they are circulative and from which they have been isolated. Yield of virus upon isolation from oats: 0.05 mg/liter sap. (Rochow *et al.*, 1971; Aapola and Rochow, 1971.)

Bean virus 1, synonym for bean common mosaic virus.

Bean common mosaic virus* (serologically related to potato virus Y group). Filamentous particles of 15×730 nm. The virus is transmitted mechanically and by aphids in a stylet-borne manner; it produces characteristic inclusions in the infected cell. (Zaumeyer and Goth, 1964.)

Bean mosaic virus 4, synonym for southern bean mosaic virus.

Bean pod mottle virus* (isometric covirus,† serologically related to cowpea mosaic virus group). Two electrophoretically different classes of 30 nm isometric particles, both containing particles of two sedimentation rates, 112 S and 91 S, in similar amounts, as well as a little of an RNA-free "top component" of 54 S. The particle weights are 7.5, 6.5, and 5.0 × 10⁶ daltons. The amounts of the two electrophoretic forms of isoelectric points pH 5.3 and 4.8 vary with age of infection. Trypsin treatment also causes the transformation of the pH 5.3 to the pH 4.8 isoelectric material, with release of certain specific amino acids. Both forms are potentially infective.

The 112 S particle is said to be infectious by itself, but greatly augmented in infectivity by addition of the 91 S species, which appears to contribute the serological, i.e., coat protein information. (Pure 112 S may not be infectious by analogy with cowpea mosaic virus.)

A_{260} (0.1%) = 8.7, the 260/280 nm absorbance ratios 1.77 and 1.70 for the 112 S and 91 S particles, respectively. The RNA contents are 37% and 30%, respectively, the molecular weights 2.5 and 2.0 × 10⁶, and A/G/U/C = 32/21/32/16 and 33/19/31/17.

The protein, as in the case of cowpea mosaic virus, consists of two components of different molecular weight occurring in similar amounts. For average amino acid composition, see Table 2.

The virus has a very narrow host range, only among legumes, some responding systemically and others with local lesions. The virus is transmitted by the leaf beetle *Ceratoma trifurcata*, as well as mechanically. The yield from soybeans is about 70 mg per liter of juice. (Moore and Scott, 1971.)

Bean yellow mosaic virus* (serologically related to pea mosaic and bean common mosaic virus, distantly related to potato virus Y group and to beet mosaic virus). Filamentous particles of 15 × 750 nm with 3.4 nm helical pitch. (Varma *et al.*, 1968.)

Bearded iris mosaic virus (similar but not serologically related to potato virus Y group). Particles of 753 nm length. (Barnett *et al.*, 1971.)

Beet curly top virus. Many strains of probably isometric 20 nm particles. Transmitted by *Circulitex tenellus.*

† See footnote on page 63.

Beet mild yellowing virus (related to beet western yellows virus).

Beet mosaic virus* (member of potato virus Y group). Filamentous particles of 13 × 730 nm. Transmitted mechanically and by aphids. (Brandes and Bercks, 1965.)

Beet western leaf roll virus (isometric, similar to barley yellow dwarf virus). Transmitted only by aphids.

Beet western yellows virus* (serologically related to turnip yellows, malva yellows, and barley yellow dwarf viruses). About 26 nm diameter isometric particles. Transmitted by aphids (*Myzus persicae*) in persistent manner. This and many biologically related yellowing viruses (barley yellow dwarf, beet mild yellowing, potato leaf roll, banana bunchy top, bean leaf roll, carrot red leaf, subterranean clover stunt, cotton anthocyanosis, filaree red leaf, malva yellows, physalis mild chlorosis, strawberry mild yellow edge, tomato yellow top, and turnip yellows) are widespread and an economically most harmful group of viruses. (Duffus, 1969, 1973.)

Beet yellow stunt virus (very similar to beet yellows virus). Semipersistent in its aphid vectors. (Hoeffert *et al.*, 1970.)

Beet yellows virus*(resembles citrus tristeza virus, but not serologically related to this or any other virus tested). Very long flexuous rods, 13.3 × 1250 nm, with 3.4 nm helical pitch and a 3.5 nm axial canal; about 13 protein subunits per turn. Unstable virus, transmitted mechanically and in semipersistent manner by aphids. (Brandes and Bercks, 1965; Duffus, 1973.)

Belladonna mosaic virus, strain of tobacco rattle virus.

Belladonna mottle virus* (serologically distantly related to turnip yellow mosaic virus, more closely to Andean potato latent virus). Isometric 27 nm particles of 5.2 × 10^6 particle weight (112 S) and top component (2.2 × 10^6?) (53 S); A_{260} (0.1%) = 8; 260/280 nm absorbance ratio 1.8; max/min 1.36 (for the mixture of particles). The RNA (37%) has a molecular weight of 2.1 × 10^6 and A/G/U/C = 23/18/27/33. The protein molecular weight is 20,300. (Bercks *et al.*, 1971.)

Betavirus 2, synonym for beet mosaic virus.

Betavirus 4, synonym for beet yellow virus.

Black locust tree mosaic virus, synonym for robinia mosaic virus.

Black raspberry (latent) virus* (multiparticle virus, serologically unrelated to many viruses tested). About 26 nm isometric particles of 98 S, 89 S, and 81 S, only the largest seemingly being infectious. The 260/280 nm absorbance ratio is 1.6. The virus has a wide host range; it is mechanically transmittable. (Converse and Lister, 1969.)

Brassica virus 1, synonym for turnip mosaic virus.

Brassica virus 3, synonym for cauliflower mosaic virus.

Brassica virus octahedron, synonym for turnip yellow mosaic virus.

Broad bean mottle virus* (BBMV) (isometric covirus similar but not serologically related to brome mosaic and cowpea chlorotic mottle virus). The icosahedral virions have a diameter of 26 nm and a particle weight of 4.8×10^6 daltons (84 S). The isoelectric point is pH 5.6; A_{260} (0.1%) = 5.4; 260/280 absorbance ratio 2.0; the buoyant density in CsCl is 1.395 g/ml.

The architecture of the particle resembles that of turnip yellow mosaic virus (with 32 morphological subunits, 20 hexamers and 12 pentamers, 180 protein molecules in all), except for the presence of a central hole 11 nm in diameter. The sensitivity of the virus to molar salt, nucleases, etc. resembles that of other members of the brome mosaic virus group.

The RNA (22%) (17 S and 10 S) is present in four components, 1.1, 1.03, 0.9, and 0.36×10^6 mol. wt., each particle presumably containing either of the two largest or the two smallest together. The three largest RNA components are essential for infectivity, thus making this a proven three-component covirus. The average A/G/U/C = 27/25/29/19.

The molecular weight of the coat protein is 21,000 daltons. It has C-terminal alanine and a probably acetylated N-terminus. For amino acid composition, see Table 2.

The virus has a very narrow host range (a few beans, peas, and clover), and can be assayed on *Chenopodium amaranticolor*. It is mechanically transmitted; no vectors are known. (Hull, 1972.)

Broad bean stain virus* (covirus, similar but probably not serologically related to cowpea mosaic virus, and echtes Ackerbohnenmosaik-Virus). The isometric particles are of 25 nm diameter, containing either 35% RNA (127 S) or 25% RNA (100 S), or none (60 S). The average A/G/U/C = 27/23/32/18. (Gibbs *et al.*, 1968.)

Broad bean true mosaic virus,* synonym for echtes Ackerbohnen-mosaik-Virus.

Broad bean wilt virus* (multiparticle virus, structurally similar to cowpea mosaic virus group, but serologically distinct; closely related or identical with nasturtium ringspot and petunia ringspot viruses). Particles of 25 nm diameter of 63 S (no RNA), 100 S (22% RNA), and 126 S (33% RNA), with 260/280 absorbance ratios of 1.32(?), 1.64, and 1.75 respectively. Only the largest RNA component appears infective. Average $A/G/U/C = 30/25/27/18$. Two proteins of 40,000 and 26,000 have been observed. The virus is aphid transmitted (nonpersistent) in contrast to the comoviruses, which have beetle vectors. (Taylor *et al.*, 1968.)

Broccoli mosaic virus, synonym for cauliflower mosaic virus.

Broccoli necrotic yellows virus* (rhabdovirus). Both bacilliform (275 × 75 nm) and bullet-shaped (270 × 66 nm) particles are observed. The average particle has 874 S and 1.19 g/ml density in potassium tartrate. The lipid-rich outer envelope is 13.5 nm thick, the protruding spikes 8.5 nm long; the pitch of the internal nucleocapsid helix is 4.5 nm. The virus contains RNA. It is ether sensitive and unstable (in all respects very similar to animal rhabdoviruses as exemplified by vesicular stomatitis virus). The virus is aphid transmitted, with a very limited host range. (Lin and Campbell, 1972.)

Brome (grass) mosaic virus* (BMV) (prototype of a group of icosahedral coviruses for which the name bromoviruses has been proposed; serologically related to cowpea chlorotic mottle virus). Three types of seemingly identical 26 nm (86 S) particles (4.6 × 10^6 daltons) of isoelectric point about pH 7.4. A_{max} (0.1%) = 5.2, the 260/280 and max/min ratios are 1.7 and 1.5. The virion is relatively heat resistant below pH 6, but swells and becomes unstable at neutrality. It is degraded by molar salt (not at 2–4 M salt concentrations), and is also sensitive to pancreatic ribonuclease, but less so to snake venom phosphodiesterase. The average density of the virus in CsCl is 1.363 g/ml. Three types of virions exist, of slightly decreasing buoyant densities on RbCl gradients, containing respectively RNA components 1, 3 + 4, and 2. The virus contains an average of 22% RNA of four types of 27 S, 22 S, and 14 S and of molecular weight 1.05, 0.95, 0.71, and 0.3 × 10^6, termed components 1–4, respectively. The latter two RNAs occur in one particle. The average $A/G/U/C = 27/28/24/20$.

All RNA components have 3′-terminal -GpCpCpCpA, the same sequence as the tobacco mosaic virus RNA. The RNA can be charged with tyrosine by appropriate enzymes. The 5′-end of the brome mosaic virus RNA components is quite heterogeneous, with 5′-unphosphorylated adenosine predominating. Thus in regard to both chain termini brome mosaic virus RNA resembles tobacco mosaic virus RNA. The RNA is about one-third as infective as the intact virus.

The protein is of molecular weight 20,000. For amino acid analysis, see Table 2. Arginine is at the C-terminus.

Virus yields are about 1 g/liter sap from barley. Few strains are known. The host range is limited, mostly grasses. Local lesions are produced on *Datura stramonium* (Jimson weed) and *Chenopodium amaranticolor*. (Lane and Kaesberg, 1971.)

BROMOVIRUS GROUP. Isometric three-component coviruses. Members: brome mosaic, cowpea chlorotic mottle, and broad bean mottle viruses.

Cabbage virus A, or cabbage black ring(spot) virus, synonym for turnip mosaic virus.

Cabbage virus B, cabbage mosaic virus, synonym for cauliflower mosaic virus.

Cacao necrosis virus (distantly serologically related to grapevine chrome mosaic virus).

Cacao swollen shoot virus* (no known relationships). Bacilliform particles of 28×125 nm (218 S). Transmitted mechanically and by several mealybug species. (Kenten and Legg, 1967.)

Cacao yellow mosaic virus* (distantly serologically related to wild cucumber mosaic and turnip yellow mosaic virus). Isometric particles of 28 nm diameter, 108 S, and a "top component" of 49 S. The 260/280 nm absorbance ratio is 1.42, the A_{max} at 264 nm, probably because the A/G/U/C of the RNA (38%) is low in guanine and high in cytosine (22/16/29/33).

The virus is mechanically transmitted. The host range is restricted. (Gibbs *et al.*, 1966.)

Cactus virus X or 1* (serologically related to potato virus X group). Flexuous filaments of 13×520 nm, containing RNA of 2.1×10^6 mol. wt. and a protein of 20,000 mol. wt. The virus is mechanically transmitted. (Brandes and Bercks, 1965.)

Cactus virus 2 (serologically related to potato virus S, M, etc.). Filaments of 650 nm.

Cantaloupe mosaic virus, synonym for watermelon mosaic virus.

CARLAVIRUS GROUP. Slightly flexuous rod viruses, longer than potex and shorter than poty viruses. Members: carnation latent, poplar mosaic, potato S, potato M, red clover vein mosaic, passiflora latent, cactus 2, chrysanthemum B, chicory blotch, pea streak, freesia mosaic, and hop latent viruses.

Carnation etched ring virus (related to cauliflower mosaic virus). Isometric particles of 47 nm diameter. Containing DNA. (Fujisawa *et al.,* 1971.)

Carnation latent virus* (prototype of carlaviruses; serologically related to potato viruses S, M, etc.). Long, slightly flexuous rods, 14×650 nm, with 3.3 nm helical pitch, a central channel, and 12 subunits per turn; 167 S and of 60×10^6 particle weight. A_{max} (0.1%) = 2.1, the 260/280 nm absorbance ratio is 1.37, the max/min ratio 1.23. The virus is relatively stable. Yields of 20–100 mg per liter sap can be obtained. The virus causes few or no symptoms, shows a narrow host range, and is transmitted mechanically as well as by aphids in a nonpersistent manner. (Varma *et al.,* 1968.)

Carnation mottle virus (no known serological relationships to many other viruses tested). Isometric particles of 28 nm diameter, 7.5×10^6 particle weight, and isoelectric point pH 5.2. The virus degrades above pH 6.2. It contains 18% RNA of molecular weight 1.4×10^6, and with A/G/U/C = 28/26/24/22. The protein has a molecular weight of 26,300. For amino acid composition, see Table 2. The yield of virus can be 600 mg/liter sap. The virus is transmitted mechanically. (Tremaine, 1970; Waterworth and Kaper, 1972.)

Carnation (Italian) ringspot virus* (similar, but not serologically related to tomato bushy stunt virus). The isometric 30 nm particle is of 135 S and 7.1×10^6 (?) particle weight. A_{max} (0.1%) = 6.5. The RNA is of 1.4×10^6 mol. wt. (21%), with A/G/U/C = 27/26/24/23. The protein molecular weight is 38,000. The virus is mechanically transmitted, possibly also by nematodes. (Kalmakoff and Tremaine, 1967.)

Carnation vein mottle virus* (serologically related to potato virus Y). The flexuous 12×790 nm particles of 144 S have A_{max} (0.1%) = 2.1; the 260/280 nm absorbance ratio is 1.15. The RNA composition is $A/G/U/C = 25/21/29/25$. The virus is transmitted by the green peach aphid *Myzus persicae* in a nonpersistent manner, as well as mechanically. (Weintraub and Ragetli, 1970.)

Carrot mottle virus (structurally similar to tomato spotted wilt virus and to the togaviridiae of animals). Spherical 50 nm diameter particles containing lipid and of 1.154 g/ml buoyant density. Persistent in aphid vectors and also mechanically transmissible. (Murant *et al.*, 1969.)

Cassava common mosaic virus* (member of potato virus X group). Filamentous particles of 15×495 nm containing 5% RNA.

Cauliflower mosaic virus* (prototype of caulimoviruses; serologically related to dahlia mosaic virus). Isometric 50 nm particles, 220 S, 28 $\times$ 10^6 in particle weight, of 1.37 g/ml buoyant density in CsCl; A_{max} (0.1%) = 7.0; the 260/280 nm absorbance ratio is 1.45.

The virus contains about 15% of circular double-stranded DNA of 4.7×10^6 mol. wt., 20 S, and effective buoyant density in CsCl of 1.702 g/ml and about 39% (G+C); its contour length is 2.3 μm; it degrades to a linear form of 18 S. The DNA renatures rapidly; it is infective. Its structure shows similarities to that of the host's DNA. The general properties of the DNA resemble those of the papilloma viruses of mammals, except for the seeming absence of the supercoiled form. These various properties suggest the presence of scissions, and of a nuclease in the preparations.

The main protein has a molecular weight of 33,000. A minor component of 68,000 may be the dimer of the same protein. The virus is quite stable; yields of 50 mg/liter sap can be obtained. The virus is transmitted mechanically as well as by aphids. It is confined mainly to cruciferous plants. *Datura stramonium* has been reported as a local lesion assay host. Infection is characterized by inclusion bodies. (Shepherd *et al.*, 1970; Russell *et al.*, 1971.)

CAULIMOVIRUS GROUP. Isometric DNA-viruses. Members: cauliflower mosaic, dahlia mosaic, mirabilis mosaic, and carnation etched ring viruses.

Celery mosaic virus* (member of potato virus Y group). Flexuous particles of 784 nm. (Brandes and Luisoni, 1966.)

Centrosema mosaic virus (member of potato virus X group). Flexuous rods, 580 nm long. (Varma *et al.*, 1968.)

Cereal striate mosaic virus (rhabdovirus). Transmitted and replicated in plant hoppers.

Cereal yellow dwarf virus, synonym for barley yellow dwarf virus.

Chenopodium mosaic and star mottle virus, synonym for sowbane mosaic virus.

Cherry chlorotic ringspot virus, synonym for prune dwarf virus.

Cherry leaf roll virus* (covirus similar but serologically not related to tobacco ringspot virus). Two types of isometric 30 nm particles (130 S, 115 S) have been observed. The 260/280 nm absorbance ratio is 1.77. The 130 S and 115 S particles contain, respectively, 43% and 40% of a 2.4 and 2.1 $\times$ 10^6 mol. wt. RNA. Highest infectivity results from a mixture of both components. The protein has a molecular weight of 54,000. (Jones *et al.*, 1973.)

Cherry (sour) necrotic ringspot virus, synonym of prunus ringspot virus.

Chicory blotch virus (probable member of carlavirus group).

Chicory yellow mottle virus (unclassified, serologically unrelated to 23 other isometric viruses). Isometric 30 nm particles, which dissociate upon freezing.

Chrysanthemum virus B* (serologically related to potato viruses S, M, etc.). Almost straight rods of 12 $\times$ 685 nm; 168 S; the 260/280 nm absorbance ratio is 1.55, the max/min ratio 1.2. Transmitted mechanically and by aphids in a nonpersistent manner.

Chrysanthemum aspermy or mosaic virus (distantly serologically related to cucumber mosaic virus and very closely to tomato aspermy virus). The isometric particles are of about 26 nm diameter. The amino acid composition is very similar to that of tomato aspermy virus. The virus is transmitted mechanically and by aphids. (Lawson and Hearon, 1970.)

Chrysanthemum stunt virus (viroid or pathogenic RNA). Similar to but not identical with potato spindle tuber virus, the infective RNA being slightly larger. Mechanically transmittable. (Diener and Lawson, 1973.)

Citrus exocortis virus (viroid or pathogenic RNA). Infectivity associated with 11 S RNA material, differing from both single-stranded and double-stranded RNA in density, enzyme susceptibility, etc., probably of molecular weight of about 80,000, and much conformational constraint. A local lesion host may be *Gynura aurantiacea;* on tomatoes bunchy top symptoms are observed similar to those produced by potato spindle tuber virus. The possibility that the two agents are identical has not been ruled out. (Semancik and Weathers, 1972.)

Citrus tristeza (or quick decline) virus* (no known relationships). Long filamentous particles of 11×2000 nm, 140 S, and 144×10^6 particle weight and 3.7 nm helical pitch. The virus contains 6% RNA and a protein of 25,000 mol. wt. It can only be transmitted by aphids in a semipersistent manner. (Price, 1966.)

Clover big vein virus, synonym for wound tumor virus.

Clover enation virus (rhabdovirus).

Clover wound tumor virus, *see* wound tumor virus.

Clover yellow mosaic virus* (serologically related to potato virus X group). Filamentous rods of 540 nm (121 S); A_{max} (0.1%) = 3.1; the 260/280 nm absorbance ratio is 1.14. The virus contains an RNA of 2.4×10^6 and a protein of 22,000 mol. wt. The virus produces cytoplasmic inclusions. (Hill and Shepherd, 1972b.)

Clover yellow vein mosaic virus (member of potato virus Y group). The particles of 12×770 nm have a 3.5 nm helical pitch. The virus produces characteristic inclusion bodies in infected cells. (Varma *et al.*, 1968.)

Cocksfoot mild mosaic virus* (serologically related to phleum mottle virus, also quite distant relationship to TYMV). Isometric particles of 28–30 nm diameter, 105 S, 5.5×10^6 dalton particle weight. The 260/280 nm absorbance ratio is 1.62. The virus contains 24% RNA of A/G/U/C = 23/27/22/28. The protein has a molecular weight of 25,000. The virus is mechanically transmitted. (Huth, 1968.)

Cocksfoot mottle virus* (not serologically related to other similar viruses tested). Isometric 30 nm particles, 118 S; 260/280 absorbance ratio = 1.60. Contains 25% RNA of 10^6 mol. wt. Transmitted by beetles. (Serjeant, 1967.)

Cocksfoot streak (or mosaic) virus* (structurally similar to potato virus Y, not serologically related to any virus tested). Flexuous 13×752 nm filaments. Transmitted by aphids.

Columbian datura virus (member of potato virus Y group).

COMOVIRUS GROUP. Isometric coviruses with two proteins. Members: cowpea mosaic, broad bean stain, bean pod mottle, echtes Ackerbohnenmosaik, red clover mottle, squash mosaic, and radish mosaic viruses.

Corium betae, synonym for beet yellow virus.

Corn mosaic virus (rhabdovirus).

COVIRUSES. Several viruses require two or more different particles carrying parts of the genome for infectivity. Those that have been well characterized, viruses related to cowpea mosaic, tobacco rattle, alfalfa mosaic, and brome mosaic, are described in terms of genome distribution in Table 3.

Cowpea aphid-borne mosaic virus (probable member of potato virus Y group).

Cowpea chlorotic mottle virus* (CCMV) (covirus, serologically related to brome mosaic virus, and able to complement it genetically). Seemingly uniform 25 nm particles (88 S) of 4.6×10^6 particle weight; isoelectric point pH 4.1; A_{max} (0.1%) = 5.8; the 260/280 nm absorbance ratio is 1.7. The virus is sensitive to molar salt and swells above pH 6.5 to a form of 78 S. Its RNA is also sensitive to pancreatic ribonuclease. The icosahedral architecture of the particle is typical, with 180 protein molecules ($T = 3$).

The virions contain 24% RNA of four different molecular weights, namely, 1.15, 1.0, 0.85, and 0.32×10^6 (23 S, 18 S, and 13 S). Thus three types of particles (one of which contains the two smallest RNA species) of very slightly different densities actually exist. Probably, as in the case of brome mosaic virus, the three largest RNA components are required for infectivity. The average A/G/U/C = 25/26/28/21.

The protein is of 19,000 mol. wt. (For amino acid composition, see Table 2.) The acetylated N-terminal sequence is approximately known up to residue 25. The C-terminus is tyrosine.

The virus has a narrow host range, including tobacco. It gives local lesions on *Chenopodium album* and *C. hybridum,* as well as soybean. It is transmitted mechanically as well as by beetles. (Bancroft, 1971; Bancroft and Flack, 1972.)

Cowpea (yellow) mosaic virus* (CPMV) (prototype for comoviruses, which all show distant serological relationship to one another;

bimodal covirus with virions containing equal amounts of two proteins). The isometric 28 nm diameter particles occur in two electrophoretic forms, each composed of two RNA-containing components of 115 S and 95 S, 7.7 and 6.0×10^6 in particle weight. Their A_{max} (0.1%) values are 10.0 and 6.2, their 260/280 nm absorbance ratios 1.67 and 1.57, respectively. There is also an RNA-free "top component" of 55 S (260/280 nm absorbance ratio 0.69). The buoyant densities in CsCl are 1.47 and 1.43 g/ml for the 115 S, 1.41 g/ml for the 95 S, and 1.30 g/ml for the "top component."

The 115 S and 95 S particles contain, respectively, 33% and 24% of RNA of 34 S and 26 S, 2.5 and 1.4×10^6 mol. wt., and with A/G/U/C = 29/33/31/17 and 28/21/32/19. These are the first plant RNAs shown to contain poly (A) sequences which are 3′-terminal and average 200 residues.

The two RNA-containing particles (or their RNAs) are required for infectivity. The two electrophoretic forms of the particles result from the splitting off of a few amino acids; the faster moving form so produced is the more infectious.

All types of particles consist of approximately equimolar amounts of two proteins of molecular weights of 42,000 and 22,000 (or 25,000 for the slower electrophoretic form). The two proteins differ in composition (see Table 2), the larger thus not representing the dimer of the smaller.

While most icosahedral plant virus and bacteriophage nucleocapsids consist of 60 triplets of identical proteins, and the animal picornaviruses of 60 tetrads composed of different proteins, the cowpea mosaic viruses seem to consist of 60 two-protein complexes.

The virus is quite stable to heat and storage. About 1 g can be obtained from 1 liter of sap when grown on cowpeas. The host range includes some nonleguminous plants; many hosts respond with local lesions, among which are *Chenopodium amaranticolor* and *Vigna sinensis*. The virus is transmitted mechanically and by certain leaf beetles. (Geelen *et al.*, 1972; Wu and Bruening, 1971.)

Cowpea strain of tobacco mosaic virus, *see* sunn hemp mosaic virus.

Cucumber virus 1 (also cucumis virus), synonym of cucumber mosaic virus.

Cucumber virus 3 and 4 (CV3, CV4) (members of tobacco mosaic virus group and distantly related to TMV; related viruses were isolated also in Czechoslovakia and Japan, among the latter the so-called cucumber green mottle mosaic viruses). The biophysical properties, including stability, of these viruses are similar to those of tobacco mosaic virus.

Proteins of different molecular weights have been reported for CV3 and CV4 (17,100 and 16,100 respectively) based on amino acid analyses (see Table 4), the latter having C-terminal alanine and probably being acetylated at the N-terminus. Both, in contrast to all other members of the TMV group, lack cysteine as well as methionine, and one contains only one tryptophan, which gives it a noticeably different UV absorption spectrum. CV3 strains are said to contain 160 or 161 amino acids, CV4 151, compared to 158 for almost all other TMV strains.

The narrow host range of these viruses, for *Cucurbitaceae* only, remained the same when CV4-RNA was reconstituted with TMV protein.

The yield of virus from cucumbers is 600 mg/liter sap. (Tung and Knight, 1972a.)

Cucumber green mottle mosaic virus (CGMMV) (strains of tobacco mosaic virus closely related to cucumber virus 3 and 4). For amino acid compositions and partial amino acid sequences of the cucumber strain (C) as well as another closely related watermelon strain (W), see Table 4 and Figure 1. For the latter no local lesion host is known. Its protein does not apparently form double disks. (Nozu *et al.*, 1971.)

Cucumber mosaic virus* (CMV) (prototype of cucumoviruses, recently recognized as representing a covirus similar to the brome mosaic virus). The 30 nm icosahedral particle of 98 S has a 5.5×10^6 particle weight; an isoelectric point of pH 4.7; A_{max} (0.1%) = 5.0; the 260/280 nm absorbance ratio is 1.65. Several strains (e.g., S, Q, Y, L) have been reported to be variously unstable to salt and pancreatic ribonuclease, strain Y being the most unstable. The virus is poorly antigenic. It contains about 18% RNA of 1.0–1.3, 0.9–1.1, 0.7–0.8, and 0.33×10^6 mol. wt. (13 S, 11 S, 8 S); average A/G/U/C = 24/23/29/23. The three largest RNA components are required for infectivity. The protein of all strains, 180 molecules of which compose a particle, has a molecular weight of 25,000. For amino acid composition, see Table 2.

The virus yield, from tobacco, is about 100 mg/liter sap. The virus has a wide host range, including tobacco and legumes. It is transmitted mechanically and by aphids, in a nonpersistent manner. Useful local lesion hosts are *Chenopodium amaranticolor* and *Vigna sinensis* (cowpea). (van Regenmortel *et al.,* 1972; Kaper and Wirt, 1972.)

Cucumber necrosis virus* (structurally similar to tomato bushy stunt virus, but not serologically related to this or any other virus tested). Isometric 33 nm diameter particles of 136 S; 9.3 × 10⁶ daltons particle weight; isoelectric point pH 3.9. Contains 18% RNA (A/G/U/C = 26/29/25/20). The protein has a molecular weight of 40,000 and lacks cysteine. The virus is transmitted mechanically and by the fungus *Olpidium cucurbitacearum.* (Tremaine, 1972.)

Cucumber yellow mosaic virus, a strain of cucumber mosaic virus.

CUCUMOVIRUS GROUP. Isometric viruses. Members: cucumber (yellow) mosaic, tomato aspermy, and peanut stunt viruses.

Cymbidium mosaic (or black streak) virus* (member of and serologically distantly related to potato virus X group). Particles of 13 × 475 nm, containing 6% RNA.

Dahlemense virus (strain of tobacco mosaic virus, Group B), *see* under tobacco mosaic virus, Table 4, Figure 1.

Dahlia (mosaic) virus* (structurally similar and serologically related to cauliflower mosaic virus). Isometric particles of 50 nm diameter (254 S); the 260/280 nm absorbance ratio is 1.5. The virus contains 16% DNA. It is difficult to transmit mechanically, is usually transmitted by aphids in stylet-borne manner. The virus forms characteristic inclusion bodies in infected cells. (Brunt, 1966b.)

Daikon mosaic virus, synonym for turnip mosaic virus.

Desmodium yellow mottle virus (serologically and physically related and similar to turnip yellow mosaic virus). The virus contains 23 S RNA compared to TYMV-RNA's 29 S, but after heating in the presence of 1% formaldehyde both viral RNAs showed about 17.5 S. Beans are good hosts for the virus. (Scott and Moore, 1972.)

DIPLORNAVIRUSES, *see* plant prototype: wound tumor virus.

Dolichos enation mosaic virus (strain of tobacco mosaic virus, not yet further classified). Preferred hosts are legumes. The virus forms mixed phenotypes with defective TMV strains. The yield is 4 g/liter sap.

Dulcamara mottle virus (distantly serologically related to turnip yellow mosaic virus). The virus contains RNA of 2.1 $\times$ 10^6 daltons, A/G/U/C = 23/17/29/31. (Bercks *et al.*, 1971.)

Echtes Ackerbohnenmosaik-Virus* (structurally similar but not serologically related to strains of cowpea mosaic virus). Stable 25 nm particles of 119 S and 98 S (probably a covirus); particle weights 7.5 and 6.1 $\times$ 10^6 daltons; A_{max} (0.1%) = 7.7; the 260/280 nm absorbance ratios are 1.81 and 1.76; RNA content 35% and 26% of 2.8 and 1.7 $\times$ 10^6 mol. wt., respectively. The average composition is A/G/U/C = 27/23/32/18. Good hosts for the virus are pea and broadbean. It is transmitted mechanically. (Paul, 1962.)

Echtes Robinienmosaik-Virus, synonym for robinia mosaic virus.

Eggplant mosaic virus* (serologically distantly related to most tymogroup members, but excluding turnip yellow mosaic virus). Isometric 30 nm diameter particles of 115 S and "top component" of 53 S. The virus contains 36% RNA of 2 to 2.5 $\times$ 10^6; A/G/U/C = 21/16/25/38. The RNA binds valine at the 3′-end under appropriate enzymatic conditions. Its protein has a molecular weight of 20,000. (Bercks *et al.*, 1971.)

Eggplant mottled dwarf virus* (rhabdovirus). Bacilliform and bullet-shaped particles (90 and 60 $\times$ 220 nm) consisting of an inner core of 50 nm diameter and a lipid-containing envelope 2–10 nm thick with 6 nm projections. The internal helical nucleocapsid at the periphery of the core is 5.5 nm thick and has a pitch of 4.5 nm. (Russo and Martelli, 1973.)

Elderberry latent virus (some structural similarity to tomato bushy stunt virus). The buoyant density of the virus in CsCl is 1.363 g/ml. The virus contains RNA of 1.55 $\times$ 10^6 mol. wt., and the main protein has a molecular weight of 40,000. (Mayo and Jones, 1973.)

Elm mosaic virus (possibly identical with cherry leaf roll virus). Polyhedral particles of 92, 65, and 45 S. The middle component (buoyant density 1.33 g/ml) is infective. (Moline *et al.*, 1971.)

Enation pea virus, synonym for pea enation virus.

Erbsenstauche-Virus, *see* red clover vein mosaic virus.

Exocortis virus, *see* citrus exocortis virus.

Fiji disease virus (diplornavirus).

Freesia mosaic virus (probable member of carlavirus group).

Golden elderberry virus, synonym for cherry leaf roll virus.

Gombo mosaic virus, *see* okra mosaic virus.

Gomphrena virus (rhabdovirus).

Grapevine chrome mosaic virus* (similar but not serologically related to tobacco ringspot virus; distantly serologically related to cacao necrosis virus). Isometric 30 nm particles of 117 S and 92 S (density in CsCl 1.486 and 1.416 g/ml). The RNA content is 40 and 31%, respectively. The virus is probably soilborne.

Grapevine fanleaf virus* (distantly serologically related to arabis mosaic virus). Isometric 30 nm particles. Transmitted mechanically and by nematodes.

Grape(vine) yellow vein virus (closely related if not identical to tomato ringspot virus). Transmitted mechanically and by nematodes. Yield from French beans 15 mg/liter sap.

Grass mosaic virus, synonym for sugarcane mosaic virus.

Green aucuba virus, *see* aucuba virus.

Henbane mosaic virus* (similar and serologically related to potato virus Y group). Rods of 14 nm diameter, either straight (in the presence of Mg^{++}) and 900 nm long, or flexuous (in the presence of EDTA) and 800 nm long; 160 S; the 260/280 nm absorbance ratio is 1.1. The composition of the RNA is $A/G/U/C = 29/26/18/27$. The protein has a molecular weight of 32,000. The yield from *Nicotiana tabacum* is about 10 mg/liter sap. The virus is transmitted mechanically, and in a nonpersistent manner by aphids. (Plumb and Vince, 1971.)

Hippeastrum mosaic virus* (similar but serologically unrelated to all potyviruses tested). Filamentous 12×750 nm rods (155 S); the 260/280 nm absorbance ratio is 1.21, the max/min ratio 1.24.

Holmes ribgrass virus (HR) (strain of tobacco mosaic virus of serologically distant relationship). The virus is much less infective than wild type virus but the RNA of both is similarly infective. HR generally gives characteristic rings upon systemic infection of *Nicotiana tabacum,* and local lesions on *Nicotiana sylvestris*. The local lesions on *Nicotiana glutinosa* and *Nicotiana tabacum* var. *Xanthi nc* are generally smaller than those given by common TMV.

The RNA shows similar properties and the same endgroups as that of wild strain TMV.

The amino acid composition indicates distant relationship, HR containing three methionine and one histidine residues, both absent from common TMV. The peptide chain is 156 rather than 158 amino acids long, the deletion having occurred near the C-terminal end. The N-terminus (AcSer-Tyr-) and C-terminus (-Pro-Ala-Thr) are the same as in common TMV, but over half of the amino acids differ along the peptide chain. The amino acid composition and sequence are given in Table 4 and Figure 1.

Hop latent virus (probable member of carlavirus group).

Hordeum mosaic virus (similar but not serologically related to ryegrass mosaic virus, structurally similar to potato virus Y group).

Hordeum virus nanescens, synonym for barley yellow dwarf virus.

Horseradish mosaic virus, synonym for turnip mosaic virus.

Hydrangea ringspot virus* (serologically related to potato virus X group). Filamentous rods of 13 × 490 nm. A_{max} (0.1%) = 3.1; the 260/280 nm absorbance ratio is 1.22. The virus contains RNA of 2.5×10^6 and protein of 22,000 mol. wt. (Varma *et al.*, 1968.)

Hyoscyamus virus I, III, synonym for henbane mosaic virus.

Iris (mild) mosaic virus* (member of potyvirus group, but not serologically related to any tested member of that group). Filamentous 12 × 760 nm particles (154 S). The 260/280 nm absorbance ratio is 1.25, the max/min ratio 1.27. The virus contains 5.5% RNA.

Kale virus (KV), strain of radish mosaic virus.

Kartoffel-K (or Rollmosaik)-Virus, identical to potato virus M.

Lactuca virus, synonym for lettuce mosaic virus.

Lettuce mosaic virus* (member of potato virus Y group). Flexuous particles of 13 × 750 nm. (Tomlinson, 1964.)

Lettuce necrotic yellows virus* (rhabdovirus). As in all plant rhabdoviruses, both bullet-shaped (66 × 227 nm) and bacilliform ("complete") particles are detectable. (It remains to be established whether both are actual *in vivo* forms, or whether one represents an artefact.) The virus is of 940 S, and shows a density in sucrose of 1.20 g/ml. The RNA is 43 S and of 4×10^6 molecular weight.

The virus is ether sensitive, due to a lipid-containing envelope, which is covered with projections 6 nm long and 6 nm apart. The virion, like all rhabdoviruses tested, contains RNA polymerase, which remains associated with the infectious nucleocapsid upon detergent treatment.

The disease is transmitted mechanically and by aphids, and both enveloped and unenveloped virus particles can be detected in various organs of the insect. The virus is obtained in low yield from *Nicotiana glutinosa*. (Randles and Francki, 1972.)

Lily mottle virus, synonym for tulip breaking virus.

Lily symptomless virus* (serologically related to carnation latent virus group, potato viruses S, M, etc.). Flexuous filaments of 18 × 640 nm (172 S) with densely staining center. The virus contains 8.3% RNA. It is transmitted mechanically and probably by *Myzus persicae;* it shows various symptoms under certain environmental conditions and in association with other viruses. (Civerolo *et al.,* 1968.)

Lucerne (or Luzerne) mosaic virus, synonym for alfalfa mosaic virus.

Lychnis virus (strain of tobacco mosaic virus, serologically related to common TMV and to the HR strain. Its amino acid composition places it in the latter group (D). (Chessin *et al.,* 1967.)

Lychnis ringspot virus (distantly serologically related to barley stripe mosaic virus). Rod-shaped particles.

Lycopersicum virus Y, synonym for tomato bushy stunt virus.

Maize chlorotic mottle virus (not serologically related to many similar viruses tested). Isometric 30 nm diameter particles.

Maize dwarf mosaic virus (similar to potato Y virus group; serologically related to sugarcane mosaic virus). The flexuous particles are of about 750 nm and 160 S and have a buoyant density of 1.3245 g/ml in CsCl. The RNA (6%) is of 39 S and has a molecular weight of 2.7×10^6; A/G/U/C = 34/20/30/16. The molecular weight of the protein is 36,000. Sorghum hybrids are used as local lesion hosts; the virus is transmitted mechanically and by aphids. (Snazelle *et al.,* 1971.)

Maize mosaic virus* (rhabdovirus). Bacilliform, not bullet-shaped, particles 48 × 240 nm, characterized by an envelop with protrusions, a membrane, a helical capsid with 4.5 nm pitch and 35 subunits per turn, as well as a dense core. A leafhopper, *Peregrinus maidis,* is the vector. (Herold and Munz, 1967.)

Maize rough dwarf virus* (diplornavirus, serologically related to rice black-streaked dwarf virus). Isometric 68 nm diameter particle (400 S) with 12 external spikes. The 45–55 nm core particle (400 S) has protrusions into (or through) the envelope. Its 260/280 nm absorbance ratio is 1.5. The virus contains double-stranded RNA. It is transmitted only by leaf hoppers, in which it is reproduced. (Lesemann, 1972.)

Malva vein clearing virus (member of potato virus Y group).

Malva yellows virus, probably identical to beet western yellows.

Melon mosaic virus, synonym for watermelon mosaic virus.

Mirabilis mosaic virus (DNA virus similar to cauliflower mosaic virus). The molecular weight of the protein is 32,000. (Brunt and Kitagima, 1973.)

Muscat melon mosaic virus, synonym for watermelon mosaic virus.

Mushroom viruses,† a poorly defined and heterogeneous group of viruses. Isometric particles of 25 to 29 nm diameter and bacilliform particles of 19 × 50 nm were described. (Dieleman-van Zaayen, 1972.)

Musk melon vein necrosis virus (serologically related to red clover vein mosaic virus). Slightly curved rods of 15 × 674 nm. (Freitag and Milne, 1970.)

Narcissus (mild) mosaic virus* (similar but serologically not related to potato virus X group). Particles of 13 × 560 nm, 114 S; the 260/280 nm absorbance ratio is 1.2; the pitch of the helix is 3.5 nm with seven subunits per turn. The RNA is of 2.4×10^6 daltons. (Wilson *et al.,* 1973.)

Narcissus yellow stripe virus* (possibly a member of potato virus Y group). Filamentous particles of 12 × 755 nm. (Brunt, 1966a.)

Nasturtium ringspot virus, probably identical with broadbean wilt virus.

Necrotic ringspot virus, synonym for prunus ringspot virus.

NEPOVIRUS GROUP. Isometric, probably coviruses. Members: tobacco

---

† For fungal viruses (penicillium, aspergillus, etc.) see Section C.

ringspot, arabis mosaic, grapevine fanleaf, raspberry ringspot, strawberry latent ringspot, tomato blackring, and tomato ringspot viruses.

Netuviruses, suggested name for tobacco rattle viruses now called tobraviruses.

Nicotiana virus 7, synonym for tobacco etch virus.

Nicotiana virus 12, 13, synonyms for tobacco and tomato ringspot viruses.

Nigerian cowpea virus (serologically distantly related to tobacco mosaic virus). Forms mixed phenotypes with defective TMV strains.

Northern cereal mosaic virus (unclassified).

Oat blue dwarf virus* (unclassified). Isometric 29 nm diameter particles (119 S). The 260/280 nm absorbance ratio is 1.63. The RNA (32 S) has a molecular weight of 2.1×10^6.

Oat necrotic mottle virus (possibly a member of potato virus Y group). Filamentous 11×720 nm particles; bluegrass is a good host; no vectors are known.

Oat red leaf virus, synonym for barley yellow dwarf virus.

Oat sterile dwarf virus (diplornavirus).

Odontoglossum ringspot virus (related to tobacco mosaic virus). *See* tobacco mosaic virus; see also Table 4.

Okra mosaic virus (serologically closely related to turnip yellow mosaic virus; probable synonym gombo mosaic virus). Particles of 106 S and 42 S ("top component"). The 3´-terminus of the RNA binds valine specifically under appropriate enzymatic conditions.

Ononis yellow mosaic virus (serologically distantly related to turnip yellow mosaic virus). Isometric particles containing 37% RNA of 2.1×10^6 daltons; A/G/U/C = 21/16/29/34. (Bercks *et al.,* 1971.)

Orchid mosaic virus, synonym for cymbidium mosaic virus.

Oryza virus, synonym for rice dwarf mosaic virus.

Pangola stunt virus (probably diplornavirus). Particles of 70 nm diameter.

Papaya (mild) mosaic virus* (member of potato virus X group).

Flexuous 530-nm-long rods; 119 S; 32×10^6 dalton particle weight; isoelectric point pH 5.3; A_{260} (0.1%) = 2.9; the 260/280 nm absorbance ratio is 1.4. The virus contains 7% RNA of molecular weight 2.2×10^6 (32 S) and A/G/U/C = 34/21/22/23. The molecular weight of the protein is 19,400. The virus is mechanically transmissible; no vectors are known. (Hiebert, 1970.)

Papaya ringspot virus* (member of potato virus Y group, serologically related to watermelon mosaic virus). Flexuous particles of 12×800 nm. (Milne and Grogan, 1969.)

Parsnip mosaic virus* (similar but serologically not related to potato virus Y group). Filaments of 14×755 nm (149 S). Transmitted by aphids. (Murant and Roberts, 1971.)

Passiflora latent virus (serologically related to potato virus S, M, etc.). Filamentous particles 650 nm long.

Passion fruit woodiness virus* (member of potato virus X group similar to bean yellow mosaic virus). The particles are 12×750 nm.

Paw paw mosaic virus (member of potato virus X group). Contains RNA of 2.2×10^6 mol. wt.

Peach ringspot virus, probably identical with prunus ringspot virus.

Peach stunt virus, probably identical with prune dwarf virus.

Peach yellow bud mosaic virus (serologically related to tomato ringspot virus).

Pea virus 1, synonym for pea enation mosaic virus.

Pea early browning virus* (strain of tobacco rattle virus). The diameter of the rods is 21 nm, their length 105 and 215 nm (210 and 286 S); their buoyant density in CsCl is 1.31 g/ml. The 260/280 nm absorbance ratio is 1.15. The molecular weights of the two RNAs are 2.5 and 1.3×10^6; that of the protein 24,000. The virus is transmitted mechanically and by nematodes. (Cooper and Mayo, 1972.)

Pea enation mosaic virus* (prototype multiparticle virus). Two types of isometric 28 nm particles, 95 S and 115 S, both infectious. The average A_{max} (0.1%) = 7.5, the density in CsCl 1.42 g/ml. The two types of particles are said to contain 18% and 28% of RNA, both particles containing 1.68×10^6 dalton RNA which is infectious (30 S), but the 115 S particle also containing a 2.24×10^6 mol. wt. RNA (34 S) and a 0.36×10^6 mol. wt. RNA (12.5 S), the latter two being not infectious. No definite synergistic effects were noted upon combining different RNA components. However, quite different results were obtained more recently (on another strain). There typical covirus relationship between a 1.6×10^6 and a 1.3×10^6 mol. wt. RNA component (5.7 and 4.6×10^6 daltons), differing in protein content (180 *vs.* 150 subunits), was reported. The average composition of the RNAs is A/G/U/C = 24/26/26/24.

The protein is of 21,800 mol. wt. For amino acid composition, see Table 2. The virus is not very stable above 50°C, and of medium stability in sap. Good yields can be obtained from peas (up to 300 mg/liter sap). The virus is transmitted mechanically and by aphids. It persists in aphids, and has been isolated from them. It has a restricted host range, but infects some nonleguminous plants. Local lesion hosts suitable for testing are *Chenopodium amaranticolor* and *C. quinoa.* (Gonsalves and Shepherd, 1972; Hull and Lane, 1973.)

Pea mosaic virus (a member of potato virus Y group, a strain of bean yellow mosaic virus).

Peanut mottle virus (similar to members of potato virus Y group, but serologically unrelated to soybean mosaic, bean common mosaic, potato Y, or tobacco etch viruses). Flexuous rods of 740 nm. The virus causes typical inclusion bodies. (Sun and Hebert, 1971).

Peanut stunt virus* (a legume-infecting strain of cucumber mosaic virus). Isometric 30 nm particles (98 S) of 6.8×10^6 particle weight; A_{max} (0.1%) = 4.8; the 260/280 nm absorbance ratio is 1.64. The particle contains 16% RNA with A/G/U/C = 26/24/29/21. (Mink, 1969.)

Pear ring pattern mosaic virus, synonym for apple chlorotic leaf spot virus.

Pea streak virus* (similar but only distantly related to red clover vein mosaic virus). Filamentous 625 nm particles (160 S). The 260/280 nm absorbance ratio is 1.34. The virus contains 5.4% RNA.

Pelargonium leaf curl virus (member of tomato bushy stunt virus group). The isometric virus is of 137 S; it contains 17% RNA of 1.5×10^6 mol. wt. Very heat and sap-storage stable. (Martelli and Russo, 1972.)

Pepper ringspot virus (strain of tobacco rattle virus). Tubular particles of two lengths, 25×54 nm and 25×199 nm, with a 4 nm axial channel. Only the long particles are infectious (presumably alone not producing stable protein-coated virus).

Pepper veinal mottle virus* (member of, but not serologically related to, potato virus Y and henbane mosaic virus group). Particles of 155 S are, depending on conditions (without or with Mg^{++}), either flexuous (12 × 770 nm) or straight (12 × 850 nm). The 260/280 nm absorbance ratio is 1.25, the max/min ratio 1.27. The RNA (5%) has A/G/U/C = 23/24/26/27. The protein molecular weight is 33,000. The virus is transmitted in a nonpersistent manner by aphids. (Brunt and Kenten, 1971.)

Petunia asteroid mosaic virus (member of tomato bushy stunt virus group).

Phaseolus virus, synonym for bean common mosaic virus.

Phleum mottle virus (serologically but not biologically related to cocksfoot mild mosaic virus).

Pisum virus, synonym for pea enation mosaic virus.

Plantain virus (rhabdovirus).

Plum pox virus* (member of potato virus Y group). Particles of 20 × 760 nm.

PM 1-6 (defective strains of TMV), *see* TMV. (Hariharasubramanian and Siegel, 1969.)

Pod mottle virus, synonym for beanpod mottle virus.

Pokeweed mosaic virus* (distant serological relationship to potato virus Y group). Flexuous particles of 13 × 776 nm. Mechanically transmitted, as well as by aphids in a nonpersistent manner. (Shepherd *et al.,* 1969.)

Poplar mosaic virus* (member of potato virus S group, but not serologically, related). Particles 675 nm long, of 165 S. (Biddle and Tinsley, 1971.)

Potato virus A* (member of potato virus Y group). Particles of 15 × 730 nm. (Brandes and Bercks, 1965.)

Potato virus E, identical with potato virus M.

Potato virus F and G, identical with potato aucuba mosaic virus.

Potato virus M* (member of carnation latent virus group, closely related to potato virus S). Particles 650 nm long. (Wetter, 1960.)

Potato virus P, synonym for potato virus A.

Potato virus S* (member of carnation latent virus group, closely related to potato virus M). Flexuous rods of 14×650 nm, with 3.4 nm helical pitch (for amino acid analysis, see Table 2). (Brandes and Bercks, 1965.)

Potato virus X* (prototype of potexvirus group; many strains, showing considerable variations). Slightly flexuous $11.5 \times 480-580$ nm rods (118–124 S), about 35×10^6 in particle weight, isoelectric point pH 4.4, 3.4 nm helical pitch, ten subunits per turn (about 147 turns). A_{max} (0.1%) = 2.97, the 260/280 nm absorbance ratio is 1.2. The virus contains 6% RNA of 2.1×10^6 mol. wt., with A/G/U/C = 34/22/21/23. Protein is of 27,000 mol. wt. (for amino acid analysis, see Table 2), but decreases in molecular weight upon storage due to protease action. It has an acetylated N-terminus and -Pro at the C-terminus. The virus is very heat and storage stable, and the yield from tomatoes can be over 1 g/liter sap. The virus is widely distributed and mechanically transmitted. It has a moderate host range and produces local lesions on globe amaranth (*Gomphena globosa*) and ornamental goosefoot (*Chenopodium amaranticolor*). (See Electron micrograph XVI.) (Tung and Knight, 1972b.)

Potato virus Y* (prototype of potyvirus group, longer particles than the potex group). Long flexuous rods 11×730 nm, with 3.4 nm helical pitch. Contains 6% RNA and a protein of 21,300 mol. wt. (for amino acid analysis, see Table 2). Most members of the potato virus Y group are quite heat sensitive and unstable in sap. They are transmitted by aphid vectors in a nonpersistent manner, as well as mechanically. The yield from tobacco is 4 mg/liter sap. Characteristic pinwheel inclusion bodies are seen in infected cells. Moderate host range, several hosts showing local lesions suitable for quantitation (*Lycium barbarium*, barberry, wolfberry, and *L. chinense*, the chinese wolfberry). (Miki and Oshima, 1972b.)

Potato acropetal necrosis virus, synonym for potato virus Y.

Potato aucuba mosaic virus* (member of, but not serologically related to, potato virus X group). Filamentous particles of 11×580 nm (130 S); A_{260} (0.1%) = 2.6; the 260/280 nm absorbance ratio is 1.1. The virus contains 5% RNA, A/G/U/C = 30/25/21/24. The protein has a molecular weight of about 23,000. The virus is aphid transmitted (*Myzus persicae*) only in the presence of other potato viruses (A or Y), as well as mechanically. (Miki and Oshima, 1972a.)

Potato calico virus, synonym for potato aucuba mosaic virus.

Potato corky ringspot virus, strain of tobacco rattle virus.

Potato interveinal mosaic virus, identical with potato virus M.

Potato latent virus, synonym for potato virus X.

Potato leaf roll virus* (similar but not serologically related to beet western yellows or barley yellow dwarf virus). Isometric particles of 24 nm diameter. Transmitted by and circulative in aphids. Can be isolated from aphids (*Myzus persicae*) and plants (*Physalis floridana*). (Peters and van Loon, 1968.)

Potato mild mosaic virus, synonym for both potato virus X and A.

Potato mop-top virus (serologically very distantly related to TMV). Straight rod-shaped particles of various lengths (mostly 250–300 nm) and same width and helical pitch as TMV. Only the longest particles are infectious. Normally fungus transmitted (*Spongospora subterranea*), but also mechanically transmittable. (Kassanis *et al.*, 1972.)

Potato paracrinkle virus, synonym for potato virus M.

Potato phloem necrosis virus, synonym for potato leafroll virus.

Potato spindle tuber virus* (prototype viroid or "pathogenic RNA"). No virus particles detected. Infectivity is associated with RNA, probably single-stranded with much base pairing, of about 80,000 mol. wt. (about 250 nucleotides long), with 3′-terminal A and a contour length of 55 nm. Larger infective "aggregates"(?) are also usually found. Narrow host range, mainly *Solanaceae,* generally showing systemic infection. *Scopolia sinensis* shows both local and systemic symptoms and has been proposed as a local lesion assay host. The virus is possibly identical to citrus exocortis virus. (Diener, 1972.)

Potato stem mottle virus, strain of tobacco rattle virus.

Potato yellow dwarf virus* (rhabdovirus). Two serotypes are known. Bacilliform 380×75 nm particles (900 S) of buoyant density in sucrose of 1.17 g/ml, and particle weight of 1100×10^6. Contains 20% lipid; 0.2% (45 S) RNA of 4.6×10^6 mol. wt., $A/G/U/C = 28/23/28/21$; buoyant density in CsCl 1.65 g/ml; and four proteins of 22,000, 33,000, 56,000 and 78,000 mol. wt. (molar ratios

1:3:3:2), the latter a glycoprotein. The 56,000 protein represents the nucleocapsid protein. It and the smallest one determine serotype specificity, the other two group specificity. (For amino acid analysis, see Table 2.) The virus is transmitted and replicated by leafhoppers. (Reeder *et al.,* 1972.)

Potato viruses A–Y, *see* after poplar mosaic virus.

POTEXVIRUS GROUP. Medium long filamentous viruses. Members: artichoke curly dwarf, cactus X, cassava common mosaic, clover yellow mosaic, cymbidium mosaic, hydrangea ringspot, narcissus mosaic, papaya mosaic, potato acuba mosaic, potato X, and white clover mosaic viruses.

POTYVIRUS GROUP. Long filamentous viruses. Members: bean common mosaic, bean yellow mosaic, beet mosaic, carnation vein mottle, celery mosaic, clover yellow vein, cocksfoot streak, Columbian datura, cowpea aphid-borne mosaic, henbane mosaic, iris mosaic, malva vein clearing, narcissus yellow stripe, pea mosaic, plum pox, potato A, potato Y, soybean mosaic, sugarcane mosaic, tobacco etch, tulip breaking, turnip mosaic, and watermelon mosaic viruses.

Prune dwarf virus* (related to tobacco streak virus). Isometric particles of 22 nm diameter; 260/280 nm absorbance ratio 1.56. (Fulton, 1968.)

Prunus (necrotic) ringspot virus* (multiparticle virus, serologically related to apple mosaic virus). Isometric particles 24 nm in diameter, of 96 and 123 S and a "top component." Labile virus, stabilized by chelating but not by reducing agents; contains 16% RNA; A/G/U/C = 25/27/27/21. The protein is of mol. wt. 25,000 (for amino acid analysis, see Table 2). (Barnett and Fulton, 1969.)

Radish mosaic virus* (covirus, member of cowpea mosaic virus group, serologically related to this as well as to beanpod mottle and squash mosaic viruses). Isometric 30 nm diameter particle. The two nucleoprotein components of isoelectric point pH 4.3 have 97 and 116 S; A_{max} (0.1%) = 9 and 11; 260/280 nm absorbance ratio 1.65 and 1.78; they contain 26 and 35% RNA of 1.3 and 2.2×10^6 mol. wt. and A/G/U/C of 29/22/30/19 and 30/25/27/18. Transmitted mechanically and by beetles.

Radish P and R viruses, synonyms for turnip mosaic virus.

Radish yellows virus, synonym for beet western yellows virus.

Raspberry ringspot (or Scottish leaf curl) virus* (covirus, similar but not serologically related to the tobacco ringspot or nepovirus group). Particles of 30 nm diameter. Three components: 130 S particles, (5.6 × 10⁶ particle weight) containing 43% RNA of 2.4 × 10⁶ mol. wt, 92 S (5.0 × 10⁶ particle weight) containing 29% RNA of 1.4 × 10⁶ mol. wt.; the 260/280 nm absorbance ratios for these two virion components are 1.78 and 1.62. Also an RNA-free "top component" of 50 S. The largest RNA component is infective, but its infectivity is potentiated by the presence of the smaller. The latter appears to contribute the serological, i.e., coat protein, information. The protein has a molecular weight of 54,000 (probably 72 molecules per particle). The virus has a wide host range; it is transmitted by nematodes. (Murant *et al.,* 1972.)

Ratel-Virus, synonym of tobacco rattle virus.

Red clover mottle virus* (covirus, serologically closely related to cowpea mosaic virus group). Isometric 30 nm particles of 60 S ("top component"), 101 S, and 127 S, the latter components containing 25% and 36% RNA. Mixed A_{max} (0.1%) = 13.0; the 260/280 nm absorbance ratio is 1.5 and 1.7, respectively. The 101 S component is not infective but greatly augments the infectivity of the partially purified 127 S component. The average A/G/U/C is 29/20/30/20. (Gibbs *et al.,* 1968.)

Red clover vein mosaic virus* (distantly serologically related to carnation latent virus group, closely related to pea streak virus). Filamentous particles of 12 × 645 nm, 160 S, isoelectric point pH 4.5; the 260/280 absorbance ratio is 1.14; 3.4 nm helical pitch, ten subunits per turn. RNA content 6.3% of A/G/U/C = 24/31/22/23. Transmitted mechanically and with low efficiency by aphids in a nonpersistent manner. (Wetter *et al.,* 1962; Varma *et al.,* 1968.)

Red currant ringspot virus, synonym for raspberry ringspot virus.

Rhabarber-Mosaik-Virus, synonym for arabis mosaic virus.

Rʜᴀʙᴅᴏᴠɪʀᴜsᴇs. Large, enveloped, lipid-containing, ether-sensitive, bullet-shaped or bacilliform viruses exemplified by the vesicular stomatitis virus of swine. They contain an RNA polymerase. Plant prototypes: wheat striate mosaic and lettuce necrotic yellow viruses.

Ribgrass mosaic virus, *see* Holmes ribgrass mosaic virus.

Rice black streaked dwarf virus (diplornavirus, related serologically to maize rough dwarf virus). (Luisoni *et al.,* 1973.)

Rice dwarf virus* (diplornavirus, similar to reoviruses of mammals and insects, as well as wound tumor virus, etc., but no known serological relationships). Isometric 70 nm particles (510 S) with dense 50 nm cores (32 capsomeres, consisting of inner and outer icosahedral shells as well as empty shells). The virions contain 12 strands of different length of double-stranded RNA (11%); average $A/G/U/C = 28/22/28/22$; they also contain RNA polymerase. Leafhoppers are persistent vectors. The virus has a narrow host range confined to the grass family and gives only systemic symptoms. (Miura *et al.*, 1966.)

Rice mosaic and stunt viruses, synonyms for rice dwarf virus.

Rice transitory yellowing virus* (rhabdovirus of no known serological relationships). Particles of 96×130 and 94×190 nm, depending on technique used. Transmitted by green leafhoppers in a persistent manner. (Chen and Shikata, 1971.)

Rice tungro (or yellow orange) virus* (unclassified). Polyhedral particles of 30–35 nm diameter, 175 S; the 260/280 nm absorbance ratio is 1.45. Contains about 11% RNA. Virus, transmitted by leafhoppers, e.g., *Nephotettix impicticeps,* is circulative and semipersistent in vector; it is comparatively stable. (Gálvez, 1968.)

Robinia mosaic virus* (unclassified). Particles of 40 nm diameter. (Schmelzer, 1967.)

Rotkleeadernmosaik-Virus, *see* red clover vein mosaic virus.

Russian winterwheat mosaic virus (rhabdovirus). Transmitted and replicated in leafhopper.

Ryegrass (streak) mosaic virus* (similar but not serologically related to wheat streak mosaic virus). Flexuous rods of 700 nm. (Varma *et al.,* 1968.)

Ryegrass streak virus, synonym for brome mosaic virus.

Sammon's opuntia virus (related to tobacco mosaic virus). Rods, 315 nm long.

Satellite tobacco necrosis virus* (small defective virus; several strains). Icosahedral particles of 17 nm diameter; 2×10^6 particle weight; 50 S; isoelectric point pH 4.3; A_{260} (0.1%) = 6.5; the 260/280 nm absorbance ratio is 1.65; contains 20% RNA of 14 S and 0.4×10^6 mol. wt. The RNA ($A/G/U/C = 28/25/25/22$) starts with (p)ppApGpU- and ends with -GpApCpUpApCpCpC(p), with partly a third phosphate on the left end (pppA-) and partly also a phosphate on the right end (-Cp), the only instance of a 3´-phosphorylated RNA chain end.

The protein has 22,800 mol. wt. (see Table 4 for amino acid analysis). Strain SV_c is of 24,900 mol. wt. No N-terminal residues have been detected, and leucine is C-terminal. Probably 72 molecules of protein compose a particle. Both ends of the peptide chain are alanine. (See Electron micrograph XV.)

The virus is replicated only in the presence of tobacco necrosis virus, with strict strain-specific relationship in regard to both satellite and helper virus. Yet the proteins of these two viruses are serologically unrelated, and no evidence for chemical or genetic relationship is available. The yield of virus is optimally 30 mg/liter sap from tobacco or French beans. (see Table 3.) (Rees *et al.*, 1970.)

Scrophularia mottle virus* (serologically distantly related to turnip yellow mosaic virus). Isometric virus of 26 nm diameter; A_{max} (0.1%) = 8; the 260/280 nm absorbance ratio is 1.79. It contains 37% RNA of 2.1×10^6 daltons, A/G/U/C = 21/16/29/34. The molecular weight of the protein is 21,600. (Bercks *et al.*, 1971.)

Severe etch virus, *see* tobacco etch virus.

Soil-borne wheat mosaic virus, *see* wheat mosaic virus.

Solanum virus 1, synonym for potato virus X.

Solanum virus 2, synonym for potato virus Y.

Solanum virus 3, synonym for potato virus A.

Solanum virus 7, 11, synonyms for potato virus M.

Sorghum red stripe virus (serologically related to sugarcane mosaic virus).

Sour cherry necrotic ringspot virus (similar to tobacco streak virus).

Sour cherry yellows virus, synonym for prune dwarf virus.

Southern bean mosaic virus 1* (prototype, serologically unrelated to other similar viruses; has three known strains). Particles of 27 nm diameter, 115 S, 6.5×10^6 in particle weight; A_{max} (0.1%) = 5.6; the 260/280 nm absorbance ratio is 1.6; density in CsCl 1.43 g/ml. Contains 21% RNA, 25 S, of 1.35×10^6 mol. wt.; A/G/U/C = 23/27/27/23. The protein is of 30,000 mol. wt., and 180 molecules build up a virion (for amino acid analysis, see Table 2). The virus is particularly stable. It has a narrow host range (leguminous species only); it is transmitted by beetles as well as mechanically. The yield from beans is about 800 mg/liter sap. Different virus strains may give local lesion and/or systemic infection on different common bean varieties. (Ghabrial *et al.,* 1967; Kaper and Waterworth, 1973.)

Sowbane mosaic virus* (serologically unrelated to many isometric viruses tested). Isometric 26 nm diameter particles with a dense core, 104 S, 6.3×10^6 particle weight, isoelectric point pH 4.4; A_{max} (0.1%) = 4.9; the 260/280 nm absorbance ratio is 1.5, the max/min ratio 1.67. The virus contains 20% RNA of 1.3×10^6 mol. wt. The composition of the RNA is A/G/U/C = 23/26/23/28. The coat protein of 19,200 mol. wt. is probably acetylated at the N-terminus and carries lysine at the C-terminus. (For amino acid analysis, see Table 2.) (Kado and Black, 1968.)

Sowthistle yellow vein virus* (rhabdovirus, structurally and biologically but not serologically related to lettuce necrotic yellows virus). Predominantly bacilliform (95×230 nm), the bullet shape being regarded by some as an artifact of the staining procedure. The virus is enveloped and carries protrusions and an internal helical capsid of 4.4 nm pitch.

The virus is aphid transmitted, and shown to replicate in the aphid *Hyperomyzus lactucae.* It cannot be mechanically transmitted. It has a narrow host range. (Peters and Kitajima, 1970.)

Soybean mosaic virus* (similar, but probably serologically unrelated to potato virus Y group). Flexuous particles 750 nm long, 193 S, containing about 6.5% RNA. (Ross, 1969, 1970.)

Spinach blight virus, synonym for cucumber mosaic virus.

Squash mosaic virus* (covirus serologically related to cowpea mosaic virus group). Three (or four) isometric components 25–30 nm in diameter have been reported. The largest particle, 118 S, 6.9×10^6 in particle weight, containing 35% RNA of 2.4×10^6 mol. wt., is infectious. The 95 S particle, 6.1×10^6 in particle weight, containing 27% RNA of 1.6×10^6 mol. wt., is probably in the pure form noninfectious. The "top component" is of 57 S (4.5×10^6 in particle weight). For the nucleoprotein components A_{max} (0.1%) = 8.7 and 6.8. The RNAs of the 118 S and 95 S components have A/G/U/C = 31/23/30/16 and 32/22/29/17, respectively. There are two coat proteins of about 22,000 and 40,000 mol. wt. The virus is seedtransmitted, as well as by certain beetles. The yield from cucumber is 0.1 g/liter sap. (Lastra and Munz, 1969.)

Steinklee-Virus, *see* pea streak virus.

Strawberry latent ringspot virus (similar to tobacco ringspot virus). Like the latter, the isometric virus is transmitted by nematodes, and characterized by inclusion bodies in the infected cell.

Strawberry vein-banding virus (possible member of cauliflower mosaic virus group). Particles of 43 nm diameter embedded in dense matrix of inclusion bodies 3–4 μm in diameter.

Sugarbeet yellows virus (unclassified, not related to potato virus Y group). Flexuous rods of 11 × 1250 nm, and helical pitch of 3.4 nm. The virus is aphid transmitted in a semipersistent manner.

Sugarcane Fiji disease virus* (diplornavirus). Isometric 60–75 nm particles. The virus is transmitted only by leafhoppers. (Francki and Grivell, 1972.)

Sugarcane mosaic virus* (serologically related to maize dwarf mosaic virus and possibly to other members of the potato virus Y group). Filamentous particles of 13 × 750 nm, 176 S, 1.3327 g/ml density in CsCl. The virus, transmitted in a nonpersistent manner by aphids, more readily infects maize and sorghum than sugarcane. (Bond and Pirone, 1971.)

Sunn hemp mosaic virus (strain of tobacco mosaic virus). Shows considerable changes in properties including amino acid composition when grown on beans as compared to tobacco (where it is identical in composition to wild type TMV); *see* under tobacco mosaic virus. (Rees and Short, 1965.)

Sweet-potato russet crack virus, related to potato virus Y.

Tabakmauche-Virus, strain of tobacco rattle virus.

Tabak-Streifen and Kräusel-Krankheit Virus, synonym or strain of tobacco rattle virus.

Theobroma virus (1 or inflans), synonym for cacao swollen shoot virus.

Tobacco etch virus* (serologically related to potato virus Y and other members of the potyvirus group). The 13 × 730 nm flexuous particles (154 S) have a density of 1.33 g/ml; A_{260} (0.1%) = 2.4; the 260/280 absorbance ratio is 1.29.

The virion contains 5% RNA of A/G/U/C = 30/23/27/20. Proteins are of 26 and 32 × 10³ mol. wt. (for amino acid analysis, see Table 2). The virus has a wide host range, similar to that of tobacco mosaic virus. For local lesion assay *Physalis peruviana* (cape gooseberry) has been used. It is transmitted mechanically and in a nonpersistent manner by aphids. The virus, like others of the potato virus Y group, stimulates the appearance of characteristic inclusion bodies (pinwheels) in the cytoplasm. (Damirdagh and Shepherd, 1970; Hiebert *et al.,* 1971.)

Tobacco mosaic virus (TMV) (prototype of tobamovirus group). TMV and its more or less closely related strains are stiff rod-shaped viruses, predominantly 300 nm long, and of uniform diameter (18 nm maximal and 15 nm minimal), of 190 S, and 40×10^6 particle weight. A_{260} (0.1%) = 2.7; the 260/280 nm absorbance ratio is 1.20; the max/min ratio is 1.15 (see Electron micrograph XIV).

The TMV rod is a helix with 2.3 nm pitch and 130 turns, each containing $16\frac{1}{3}$ protein subunits (49 per 3 turns, the repeat unit). Thus the total number of protein molecules is 2130. The RNA content is 5%, its molecular weight 2×10^6, A/G/U/C = 30/25/26/19. The RNA forms a helix inside the protein helix, the diameter of the RNA helix being 4 nm, that of the protein shell 2–18 nm. The empty central canal is 4 nm in diameter. Three nucleotides are bound to each protein molecule, probably at two arginines and a lysine, the total number of nucleotides being therefore 6390. The buoyant density of TMV RNA in Cs_2SO_4 is 1.640 g/ml. TMV RNA lacks methylated bases and contains no poly (A) sequences.

The RNAs of several strains of TMV have been subjected to some structural analyses which have shown that the 5′-end is unphosphorylated and predominantly adenosine, followed by G and U, but apparently not the same for all molecules. (Similar heterogeneity was found for the 5′-end of all components of brome mosaic virus RNA). In contrast, the 3′-end is uniformly -GpCpCpCpA, and this is true for other strains and mutants to the extent that it was investigated. Upon degradation of TMV RNA by the guanine-specific T1 ribonuclease, the six largest oligonucleotides were isolated, characterized by containing only one (terminal) guanine residue. They are one of about 69 residues, two of 26 residues, and three of 15–18 residues. The largest of these was found to vary in length and composition among certain not closely related strains of TMV (Dahlemense, U2). Through controlled progressive stripping of the protein from the TMV rod, the location of the three largest (ω, ψ_1, and ψ_2) on the RNA chain could be approximately ascertained as within 180, 380, and 2800 bases from the 3′-end of the RNA.

Through chemical modification of the RNA *in situ* in the virus rod or in the free state, particularly with nitrous acid, which transforms cytidine to uridine and adenosine to inosine residues, mutations can be produced which are detectable by altered symptoms on test plants and which may or may not be associated with coat protein alterations. Over 1000 chemically produced mutants have been studied in this and other respects.

The protein coat consists of 2130 molecules of about 17,500 mol. wt., made up generally of 158 amino acids, although the Holmes ribgrass strain has 156 amino acids in its protein coat, and various interrelated cucumber viruses are said to contain 160, 161, and 151 residues and have molecular weights of 17,000 and 16,100, a surprising difference in view of the fact that serological relationship between these viruses (CV3 and CV4) and TMV has been demonstrated (see Table 4).

Natural virus isolates resembling TMV in its quite characteristic shape and size have generally been found to be serologically related to the prototype, common TMV as isolated by W. M. Stanley at Princeton in 1935. These serological cross-reactions have indicated close, intermediate, and distant relationships. The coat proteins of prototypes of these strains have been analyzed for amino acid composition, and in four cases for complete amino acid sequence, and these analyses have borne out the various stages of relatedness. On the basis of their showing progressive increases or decreases in the rarer amino acids they can be grouped as A-I (see Table 4), with 4, 5, 6, 7, 7, and 4 tyrosines; 0, 1, 2, 3, 3, and 0 methionines, etc. Group A contains many strains differing by 0–3 amino acid replacements from the common, wild type, vulgare, or U1 strain; group B contains the Dahlemense and tomato atypical mosaic virus Y strain; group C contains the U2 and tomato atypical mosaic virus G strain; group D contains the Holmes ribgrass virus (HR, U8); group E contains the odontoglossum ringspot virus; and groups F–I contain the cucumber mosaic 3 and 4 and related Japanese viruses. While in tyrosine and methionine content group F cucumber viruses 3 and 4 resemble the wild type TMV, they are actually very different (lacking the cysteine and carrying C-terminal alanine), and the strain relationship of this group to the TMV group has often been questioned. Each of the groups A–H, excepting D, contains two or more members isolated at different times and places and differing by 0–3 amino acid replacements.

Comparison of the amino acid sequences of members of groups A–D also shows progressively greater numbers of amino acid replacements. Thus common TMV and HR differ by over 80 of the

158 or 156 residues per chain. Yet certain dipeptide and longer segments of the chain remain unaltered in all strains that have been analyzed and/or sequenced. These are cysteine (residue 27), Glu-Phe-Glu (34–36), Glu-Phe (47–48), Arg-Phe-Pro (61–63), Val-Tyr (69–70), Pro-Leu (78–79), Ala-Leu (82–83), Phe-Asp-Thr-Arg-Asp-Arg-Ile-Ile-Glu (87–95), Arg-Val-Asp-Ala-Thr-Val-Ala-Ile-Arg (113–122), Glu-Leu (131–132), Phe-Glu (144–145), and the C-terminal heptapeptide (Trp-Thr-Ser-Ala-Pro-Ala-Thr) (see Figure 1).

All strains of TMV show "protected" ends in the sense that they are particularly resistant to exopeptidases. Most of them have N-terminal acetyl groups, and the exception, U2, has proline at that end. The proline in third position from the C-terminus in all strains fulfills a similar role, allowing carboxypeptidase to remove no more than the terminal threonine or serine.

The chemically produced mutants or those observed to occur spontaneously usually show only one, two, or rarely three amino acid replacements, not next to one another. Viable mutants have not shown exchanges in the areas found immutable in the natural strains related to TMV which were discussed above. Certain mutants are characterized by their protein being functional (i.e., able to aggregate around the RNA to form rods) only below certain temperatures, i.e., they are temperature-sensitive mutants. Among those are two (one spontaneous, called flavum, and one nitrous-acid-produced, Ni 118) with replacements at residues 19 (Asp→Ala) and 20 (Pro→Leu), respectively. In these the coat protein was found more sensitive to heat denaturation *in vitro* than is wild type TMV protein. Other temperature-sensitive mutants show no amino acid exchanges in the coat protein.

Other mutants are characterized by proteins which are defective and nonfunctional at all temperatures (strains PM 1–6), while retaining some aggregating tendency that made their isolation possible. The amino acid exchanges in these proteins, to the extent that they were allocated, appear no more drastic, qualitatively or quantitatively, than those in functional proteins, except that in the case of PM 2 one of two exchanges is a Glu→Asp replacement occurring in an "immutable" region (residue 95).

Two TMV strains isolated from leguminous plants (cowpea and sunn hemp) showed considerable differences in properties including amino acid compositions when grown on beans as compared to tobacco (12 exchanges, no cysteine, only 1 lysine, 1 tryptophan, 8 tyrosines). Grown on tobacco, the sunn hemp mosaic virus is identical to wild type in composition and the cowpea strain shows 1 or 2 exchanges. (Lauffer and Stevens, 1968; Mundry and Priess, 1971.)

Tobacco necrosis viruses* (TNV) (prototype virus). Several groups of strains of more or less distant serological relationship have been combined under this name, largely on the basis of biological and physical similarities. Typical TNV particles are isometric and of 26–28 nm diameter, 120 S, about 7×10^6 dalton particle weight; isoelectric point pH 4.5; A_{260} (0.1%) = 5.3; the 260/280 nm absorbance ratio is 1.7; buoyant density in CsCl 1.399 g/ml (see Electron micrograph XV).

TNV contains about 19% RNA (14 S) of 1.3×10^6 mol. wt. The A/G/U/C composition has been reported for the Urbana strain as 29/23/24/24, for the U. C. Davis AC 36 strain as 26/24/28/22, and for a Rothamstead isolate as 28/25/25/22, data which suggest that these are not strains of the same virus.

Protein molecular weight determinations, in part based on minimal molecular weight histidine analyses, have ranged from 23,000 to 33,000, but it appears that the higher value is more nearly correct. However, marked amino acid compositional differences have also been observed (see Table 4).

AC 36 has no detectable N-terminus, while that of the Rothamstead (or A) and Urbana strains is alanine; the C-terminal is isoleucine and -Ser-Val-Val-Met, respectively. These TNV strains, or rather these chemically and serologically not closely related viruses, support different satellite tobacco necrosis strains (e.g., AC 36 supports SV_c).

"Tobacco necrosis virus" is also of greatly variable stability upon heating and storage, as well as yield from tobacco (10–100 mg/liter sap). The host range is wide, the infection almost always localized, and usually tested on tobacco or beans. These viruses can be transmitted mechanically, but are normally soil-borne, the fungus *Olpidium brassicae* representing the vector. (Kassanis *et al.,* 1972.)

Tobacco rattle virus* (prototype of tobraviruses, rod-shaped viruses of two characteristic lengths; the only known group of coviruses with one defectively infective component). Three serotypes have been described: A, HSN, PRN; ORE, mild; and most distantly related, CAM. The pea early browning virus (SP 5) also is serologically related to these viruses. The diameter of the rods is about 22 nm, the pitch of the helix 2.5 nm. The long rod varies from 180 nm to 210 nm in length for different strains (300 S, 46–50 $\times$ 10^6 particle weight). The short rod ranges from 52 nm to 110 nm in different strains (12–29 $\times$ 10^6 particle weight). A_{260} (0.1%) = 3.0, and the 260/280 nm absorbance ratio is 1.15.

The RNA (5%) in the long rod is of 2.5 $\times$ 10^6 mol. wt. (26 S), that of the short rod (12–20 S) proportionately smaller (0.7, 1.0, 1.3 $\times$ 10^6 for CAM, PRN, and SP 5 of the pea early browning virus). Both RNA chains of the CAM isolate terminate with -GpCpCpC, but their nucleotide sequences are not similar, possibly excepting a 500 nucleotide segment.

The single type of protein covering both long and short rods has a molecular weight of 20,000–29,000 for different strains and investigators (e.g., 28,500 for CAM and PRN, 24,000 for SP 5). Amino acid analyses support the above serological grouping of strains; the C-terminus is proline.

Tobacco rattle viruses represent a class of coviruses in which the larger piece of RNA is seemingly sufficient for all aspects of the infection process except coat protein synthesis. Thus the large component or its RNA cause typical infection but not the formation of stable virus particles. The mixture of long and short rods represents the complete genome (Table 3).

The tobacco rattle viruses are quite heat and storage stable; yields of 100 mg/liter sap (from *Nicotiana clevelandii*) are typical. The viruses are transmitted mechanically and by nematodes (*Trichodorus* spp.); they have a wide host range and tend to give considerable necrosis on infected leaves. They are conveniently tested on common beans. (Sänger, 1969; Cooper and Mayo, 1972; Minson and Darby, 1973.)

Tobacco ringspot (#2) virus* (prototype of a group of multiparticle isometric viruses, possibly coviruses; other members: raspberry ringspot virus, definitely a covirus; the name nepoviruses has been proposed for these viruses).

Isometric particles of 29 nm, 92 S and 127 S, of 4.9 and 5.7 $\times$ 10^6 particle weight; A_{260} (0.1%) = 10; the 260/280 nm absorbance ratios are 1.37 and 1.88. A "top component" of 3.3 $\times$ 10^6 particle weight (53 S) lacking RNA is also observed.

The RNA of the two components is 24 S and 32 S, 27% and 40%, respectively, of 1.2 and 2.2 $\times$ 10^6 mol. wt. The average RNA composition is A/G/U/C = 23/24/30/22. The larger virus particle or its RNA component is sufficient for infectivity, but the infectivity is increased by the presence of the smaller RNA component. Thus this probably represents another covirus system, and it remains to be established whether the infectivity in the larger component is due to residual presence of traces of the smaller component. The coat protein is of 28,000 mol. wt.

The virus is moderately heat stable and quite stable in sap; the yield from cowpeas is about 25 mg/liter sap. The virus is mechanically transmissible, and naturally is transmitted by nematodes, in which it persists for long periods of time; it has a wide host range. Infection leads to the appearance of characteristic tubular inclusion bodies containing the virus.

Multiple smaller satellite-like particles have been reported to accompany the ST strain of tobacco ringspot virus. One satellite strain (SL) has also been described with an RNA of molecular weight 86,000 (7 S), occurring multiply in the particle. Since this noninfective particle contains typical tobacco ringspot virus protein, it bears no relationship to the satellite-helper system of tobacco necrosis virus. (Kaper and Waterworth, 1973.)

Tobacco streak virus* (covirus system, similar but serologically unrelated to Tulare apple mosaic virus). Particles of three sizes (about 28 nm) sedimenting with 90 S, 98 S, and 113 S, all containing RNA. This appears also to be a covirus system, with the infectivity of the 113 S particle being greatly potentiated by the presence of the 98 S particle and maximum infectivity resulting from the presence of all three components. A_{260} (0.1%) = 5.1, the average 260/280 nm absorbance ratio is 1.56. A/G/U/C = 25/25/30/20.

Several RNA components have also been reported (1.3, 1.06, 0.78, and 0.36 $\times$ 10^6), but degradation during the phenolation has not been ruled out. The protein has a molecular weight of 28,500 daltons. The virus has a very wide host range, with common bean serving as one of several local lesion hosts. It is generally transmitted mechanically. (Lister and Bancroft, 1970.)

Tobacco vein-banding (or veinal necrosis) virus, probably identical to potato virus Y.

Tobamovirus group. Stiff rod-shaped viruses of 300 nm length. Members: tobacco mosaic (U1), aucuba mosaic, Dahlemense and U2, tomato (atypical) mosaic, odontoglossum, dolichos enation mosaic, cucumber 3 and 4, cucumber green mottle mosaic, Holmes ribgrass, sunn hemp mosaic, and Sammon's opuntia viruses.

Tobravirus group. Rod-shaped coviruses with one defective-infective component. Members: tobacco rattle and pea early browning viruses. (Cooper and Mayo, 1972.)

Tollkirschen-Scheckungs-Virus, synonym for belladonna mottle virus.

Tomato aspermy virus* (closely related to a chrysanthemum aspermy virus and distantly serologically related to cucumber mosaic viruses). Isometric 28 nm particles, 99 S, of 5.3×10^6 dalton particle weight, with a 260/280 nm absorbance ratio of 1.75. Contains 18% RNA of A/G/U/C = 26/24/29/21. The protein of 26,000 daltons differs in only four amino acid residues from that of chrysanthemum aspermy virus. (Stace-Smith and Tremaine, 1973.)

Tomato atypical mosaic virus (yellow and green = Y and G strains; strains of tobacco mosaic virus, belonging to class B and C respectively, one amino acid exchange from Dahlemense and U2 strain, respectively, see Table 4). The Y strain from tomatoes is very similar to many other tomato isolates of TMV; the G strain isolated from it on tobacco is no longer able to infect tomatoes. (Wang and Knight, 1967.)

Tomato black ring virus* (covirus, similar but not serologically related to tobacco ringspot virus). Isometric 30 nm particles of 55 S (top component), 97 S, and 121 S, the latter containing 28% and 38% of RNA, respectively, of molecular weights 1.5 and 2.5×10^6; also an 0.5×10^6 "satellite RNA." Only the two larger RNAs potentiate one another in infectivity.

The virus is nematode transmitted, like tobacco ringspot virus, and shows the same characteristic inclusion bodies. (Murant *et al.*, 1973.)

Tomato bunchy top virus, synonym for potato spindle tuber virus.

Tomato bushy stunt virus* (prototype of tombusviruses characterized by unequal amounts of two coat proteins; structurally very similar to turnip crinkle virus). Icosahedral particles with a dense core; 31 nm diameter, 132 S, 9×10^6 particle weight; isoelectric point pH 4.1; A_{260} (0.1%) = 4.5; the 260/280 nm absorbance ratio is 1.64. The virus contains 17% RNA of mol. wt. 1.5×10^6, A/G/U/C = 26/28/26/21.

The protein coat consists of 180 molecules of a protein of molecular weight 40,000 and 12 molecules of molecular weight 28,000, as well as possibly one molecule of molecular weight 80,000—two singular features for plant viruses.

The virus is built up of 90 morphological subunits, arranged in the dimer positions of a $T = 3$ icosahedral lattice. These units form

12 rings of five and 20 rings of six of the 40,000 dalton protein molecules. The 12 pentamers probably carry the second protein at the apices. In this regard bushy stunt virus may resemble ϕX 174 (where the 12 microtails are more complex), while the presence of one mole of another component suggests a maturation factor of the type occurring in the RNA of phages, although the possibility of this being an RNA polymerase must also be considered. The main protein has probably an acetylated N-terminus and leucine at the C-terminus (for amino acid analysis, see Table 2).

The virus is very heat stable (85–90°C), and also stable in sap; its yield is about 0.1 g/liter sap. The virus is mechanically transmissible. (Butler, 1970.)

Tomato etch virus, probably identical with tobacco etch virus.

Tomato fernleaf virus, synonym for cucumber mosaic virus.

Tomato mosaic viruses (strains of tobacco mosaic virus).

Tomato ringspot virus* (physically and biologically similar but serologically not related to tobacco ringspot or other similar viruses). Icosahedral 28 nm particles of 119 S and 127 S (about 5.6 $\times$ 10^6 particle weight), as well as a 3.2 $\times$ 10^6 (53 S) "top component." Isoelectric point pH 4.1; A_{260} (0.1%) = 10; the 260/280 nm absorbance ratio is 1.8. The virus contains 40% RNA (31 and 33 S) of about 2.5 $\times$ 10^6 mol. wt.; A/G/U/C = 23/26/29/22. The protein is of 24,000 mol. wt. (for amino acid composition, see Table 2). The virus is transmitted by nematodes as well as mechanically; it has a very wide host range, most hosts showing both local and systemic symptoms. The yield from cucumber cotyledons is only 2.5 mg/kg. (Tremaine and Stace-Smith, 1968.)

Tomato spotted wilt virus* (singular prototype of many strains with some similarities to, and some differences from, togaviruses). Pleomorphic 70–90 nm particles with lipid-containing envelope with 5 nm projections (540 S). Composition: 20% lipid, 7% carbohydrate, and 5% RNA of 9.5 $\times$ 10^6 mol. wt., and the unusual composition A/G/U/C = 35/38/19/9. No helical nucleocapsid has been seen. The proteins are of 84, 50, and 29 $\times$ 10^3 mol. wt., all glycoproteins, and the smallest of these is associated with the nucleocapsid. These viruses are quite unstable to heat and storage, and the yield is only 20 mg/liter sap (*Nicotiana glutinosa*). They show a wide host range. They are transmitted by thrips (in which they persist for a long time), as well as mechanically. (Francki and Grivell, 1970.)

Tomato top necrosis virus, member of tobacco ringspot virus group.

TOMBUSVIRUS GROUP. Isometric two-protein viruses. Members: tomato bushy stunt virus, artichoke mottle crinkle, carnation Italian ringspot, pelargonium leaf curl, petunia asteroid mosaic viruses.

Trespenmosaik-Virus, synonym for brome mosaic virus.

Trifolium virus 2, synonym for red clover vein mosaic virus.

True broad bean mosaic virus, *see* echtes Ackerbohnenmosaik-Virus.

Tulare apple mosaic virus* (multiparticle, possibly covirus, similar but not serologically related to tobacco streak virus). Isometric 33 nm diameter (?) particles of 91 S and 85 S, only the larger seemingly being infective. The 260/280 nm absorbance ratio is 1.36. The average composition of the heterogeneous RNA (12%) is A/G/U/C = 24/24/31/21. The protein has a molecular weight of 19,000 (for amino acid analysis, see Table 2).

　　The virus is quite unstable. It is transmitted mechanically. (Barnett and Fulton, 1969.)

Tulip Augusta disease virus, synonym for tobacco necrosis virus.

Tulip breaking virus* (distantly serologically related to potato virus Y group, particularly henbane mosaic virus). Filaments of 14×740 nm. The virus is transmitted by aphids in a nonpersistent manner.

Tulip mosaic virus, synonym for tulip breaking virus.

Turnip virus (HZ), strain of radish mosaic virus.

Turnip crinkle virus* (structurally very similar to tomato bushy stunt virus with two coat proteins, but not serologically related to any virus tested). Icosahedral particles of 29 nm diameter characterized by a dense core; 128 S; particle weight $8-9 \times 10^6$. The 260/280 nm absorbance ratio is 1.48, the max/min ratio 1.27.

　　The virus contains 17% RNA of molecular weight 1.5×10^6 and A/G/U/C = 26/28/22/24.

　　Two coat proteins have been detected, i.e., 180 molecules of molecular weight 40,000 and 12 of molecular weight 28,000 daltons, as well as a small amount of a protein of molecular weight 80,000. (For amino acid composition of the major components, see Table 2.)

The virus has a wide host range; it is transmitted mechanically and by flea beetles. (Butler, 1970.)

Turnip mosaic virus* (member of the potato virus Y group). Flexuous 720-nm-long particles. Contains 5% RNA of 3.5 × 10^6 mol. wt., A/G/U/C = 35/22/21/22. The protein has a molecular weight of 26,000. The virus is transmitted mechanically and in a nonpersistent manner by aphids. (Hill and Shepherd, 1972a.)

Turnip rosette virus* (unclassified). Isometric 28 nm diameter particle (112 S). The 260/280 nm absorbance ratio is 1.56, the max/min ratio 1.30. The composition of the RNA is A/G/U/C = 26/25/27/22; the protein has a molecular weight of 27,000.

Turnip yellow mosaic virus* (prototype for tymoviruses; distantly related serologically to wild cucumber mosaic and cacao yellow mosaic virus). Isometric 28 nm particles of 117 S and 5.6 × 10^6 dalton particle weight. The architecture of this and many structurally similar icosahedral viruses is based on 32 capsomeres, 20 hexamers and 12 pentamers (180 protein molecules). The RNA is folded into intimate contact with all capsomeres (see Electron micrograph XVI).

Besides the 117 S, there also exist small numbers of particles of lesser density due to lower RNA content, as well as many RNA-free "top component" particles (3.6 × 10^6 daltons, 54 S).

The typical virus has an isoelectric point pH 4.0; A_{260} (0.1%) = 9.6 (0.96); the 260/280 nm absorbance ratio is 1.51 (0.81); density 1.42 (1.29). (The values for the RNA-free "top component" are given in parentheses.)

The typical particle contains 34% RNA of molecular weight 1.9 × 10^6, and A/G/U/C compositions for two groups of strains as follows: 22/17/22/38 and 21/17/21/42 (note the high cytidine content). The RNA starts (at the 5′-end) predominantly with ApPy- and terminates with -CpC; valine is bound specifically by aminoacyl linkage at the 3′-terminus under appropriate enzymatic conditions apparently involving ATP (TYMV-RNA-Cp-Cp-A-valine).

The protein consists of 189 amino acid residues (see Table 2), the sequence of which is known (Fig. 2). It contains all amino acids, including four cysteine residues. The virus is comparatively heat and storage stable. It is obtained in yields of up to 0.5 g/liter sap from its best systemic host, chinese cabbage. Its host range is rather narrow and no good local lesion host is known. The virus is mechanically transmitted, as well as naturally by flea beetles. (Peter *et al.,* 1972; Kaper and Waterworth, 1973.)

Turnip (mild) yellows virus (close serological relationship with beet western yellows virus). (Duffus and Russell, 1972.)

TYMOVIRUS GROUP. Members: turnip yellow mosaic, wild cucumber mosaic, belladonna mottle, cacao yellow mosaic, Andean potato latent, dulcamara mottle, eggplant mosaic, ononis yellow mosaic, and scrophularia mottle viruses.

U1–U8, strains of tobacco mosaic virus, U1 is the wild type; U4 the masked strain also belonging to group A; U2 is a mild strain belonging to group C; U8 is the Holmes ribgrass strain (group D); U3 and U5–U7 have not yet been chemically characterized. (Siegel and Wildman, 1954.) (*See* tobacco mosaic virus; *see also* Table 4, Figure 1).

VIROIDS. Group of infective nonparticulate agents, pathogenic RNA. Members: potato spindle tuber, citrus exocortis, etc. viruses.

Watermelon mosaic virus (1)* (serologically related to papaya ringspot and muskmelon vein necrosis viruses, and structurally to other members of the potato virus Y group).Filaments 750 nm long; the virus is transmitted by aphids in a nonpersistent manner, as well as mechanically. Only *Cucurbitaceae* are hosts. (Milne and Grogan, 1969.)

Weidelgrasmosaik-Virus, synonym for brome mosaic virus.

Wheat viruses 1, 3, synonym for wheat mosaic virus.

Wheat viruses 6, 7, synonym for wheat streak mosaic virus.

Wheat mosaic virus* (some similarity to tobacco rattle and barley stripe mosaic virus, but not serologically related to any virus tested). Two lengths of stiff rod-shaped particles with hollow center, 20 × 154 and 20 × 295 nm (173 S and 212 S). The latter is infective but may not be free of shorter rod particles. A_{260} (0.1%) = 3.1, the 260/280 nm absorbance ratio is 1.20. The RNA (about 5%) is of 0.95 and 1.84 × 10^6 dalton mol. wt. (24 S and 33 S), and the larger is infective. (The question arises: does it lead to complete protein-coated virus?)

The virus has a narrow host range; it is soil-borne and transmitted by fungi (e.g., *Polymyxa graminis*), as well as mechanically. (Gumpf, 1971.)

Wheat soil-borne mosaic virus, * *see* wheat mosaic virus.

Wheat streak mosaic virus* (structurally but not biologically similar to potato virus Y group, but no serological relationship demonstrated even to the most biologically similar viruses, agropyron mosaic, ryegrass mosaic, and hordeum mosaic viruses).

Flexuous rods of 15×700 nm; 165 S; A_{260} (0.1%) = 2.7; the 260/280 nm absorbance ratio is 1.37. Contains 40 S RNA of 2.8×10^6 mol. wt.

The virus is mechanically transmitted, as well as by a mite (*Aceria tulipae*). The yield upon isolation from wheat is about 8 mg/liter sap. (Brakke and Van Pelt, 1970.)

Wheat striate mosaic virus* (rhabdovirus) (American isolates described in more detail than Australian or European ones, giving similar symptoms; no serological relationships demonstrated).

The particles are bacilliform, 240×75 nm, as observed in sections, and consist of two types of bullet-shaped particles of 270×75 nm and 400×75 nm, as well as smaller fragments when isolated. Upon purification, the virion (900 S) is covered by a membrane. A_{260} (0.1%) = 3.1; the 260/280 nm absorbance ratio is 1.25. The particles contain 24% lipids of all types and 3% carbohydrate. The RNA (5%) has A/G/U/C = 20/27/29/24. (Lee, 1968.)

White clover mosaic virus* (distantly serologically related to potato virus X). Filamentous rods, 13×480 nm (112 S); the isoelectric point is pH 4.5; A_{260} (0.1%) = 3.6; the 260/280 nm absorbance ratio is 1.2. The particles have a helical pitch of 3.4 nm, with 11 subunits per turn and an axial canal of 3.5 nm diameter. The virus contains 6% of about 3.0×10^6 mol. wt. RNA, A/G/U/C = 32/16/26/27. (Hill and Shepherd, 1972b.)

The protein of molecular weight 23,600 has a blocked N-terminus and arginine at the C-terminus. The virus has a narrow host range with local lesion response predominating. The virus is mechanically transmitted. (Tung and Knight, 1972b.)

Wild cucumber mosaic virus* (distantly serologically related to turnip yellow mosaic virus). The 28 nm particles consist, like those of turnip yellow mosaic virus, of typical virus, "top component" (53 S), and smaller amounts of intermediate components (e.g., 63 S). The infective particle (119 S) is of about 6×10^6 particle weight, with isoelectric point pH 6.6. It contains 35% RNA of 2.4×10^6 mol. wt., A/G/U/C = 17/16/26/41. This RNA is infectious, but not the 11% RNA in the 63 S component. The protein is of 23,000 mol. wt. (for amino acid analysis, see Table 2).

The virus has a narrow host range, excluding cucumber (*Cucumis sativus*), but including watermelon, squash, pumpkin, and wild cucumber. It is transmitted mechanically and by flea beetles. (Symons *et al.,* 1963.)

Wisconsin pea stunt virus, synonym for red clover vein mosaic virus.

Wound tumor virus* (prototype diplornavirus, structurally similar to reoviruses of animals, cytoplasmic polyhedrosis virus of insects, and the following plant viruses: rice dwarf, maize rough dwarf, sugarcane Fiji disease viruses. However, no serological relationship has been established among any of these).

The icosahedral particles have a diameter of 70 nm, 514 S, and 68×10^6 dalton particle weight. The nucleocapsid represents a dense central core of about 40 nm diameter. The particle probably consists of two shells of 92 morphological subunits (80 hexamers and 12 pentamers = 540 protein molecules). The 260/280 nm absorbance ratio is 1.55, the max/min ratio 1.16; A_{260} of 1.0 corresponds to 10^{12} virions/ml.

The virus contains about 20% of double-stranded RNA, occurring in 12 segments of molecular weights 2.8, 2.3, 2.08, 1.72, 1.08, 1.00, 0.76, 056, 054, and 0.32×10^6, amounting to 15.1×10^6 daltons. The average composition is 38% (G+C). The 3′-ends of all RNA double strands are one U and one C. The isolated RNA is not infective.

The four major proteins of the virion are of molecular weight 150, 122, 63, and 44×10^3 daltons, corresponding to the information content of four of the above RNA species. The virus also contains an RNA polymerase.

The virus is transmitted by and replicated in *Agallia* leafhoppers. It has a moderately wide host range, causing root and more rarely stem tumors in clover and many dicotyledonous plants. No local lesion hosts are known. Cell monolayer cultures from *Agallia constricta* provide the best assay. (Lewandowski and Traynor, 1972.)

Yellow aucuba virus, *see* aucuba virus.

Yellow bean mosaic virus, *see* bean mosaic virus.

Yellow cucumber mosaic virus (related to cucumber mosaic virus) (at least six strains).

Zea virus, *see* maize mosaic virus.

TABLE 2

Amino Acid Composition of Plant Virus Coat Proteins*

Virus	Asp	Thr	Ser	Glu	Pro	Gly	Ala	Cys	Val	Met	Ile	Leu	Tyr	Phe	Lys	His	Arg	Trp	Total number (or mol. wt.)
Alfalfa mosaic 425	21	13	15	20	17	17	20	3	13	3	5	21	4	18	14	7	11	2	224
Bean pod mottle (average of 2 proteins)	21	14	18	17	13	21	14	5	15	7	12	18	2	11	9	3	6		>201
Broad bean mottle	13	10	17	17	8	11	20		20	2	6	17	4	6	14	2	12		>185
Brome mosaic	10	11	14	17	6	10	32	1	17	3	9	15	5	5	13	4	14	3	180
Carnation mottle	23	24	18	20	15	19	20	3	22	6	12	17	6	9	16	1	12	1	244
Carnation ringspot	34	37	37	23	20	20	24	3	36	7	16	26	16	12	14	2	16	4	347
Cowpea chlorotic mottle	10	16	15	17	7	9	26	2	19	1	7	16	5	4	12	2	8	4	183
Cowpea mosaic S	23	13	13	16	21	11	15	4	14	5	11	20	6	12	15	4	9	6	197
L	37	31	30	26	18	29	21	12	24	9	20	30	11	4	15	11	17	11	372
Cucumber mosaic	22	13	24	15	14	12	13	0	16	6	12	20	8	4	14	3	18	1	215
Cucumber necrosis	46	31	32	24	23	32	41	0	33	1	20	33	12	20	16	3	17	7	391
Pea enation mosaic	21	13	16	14	11	21	17	3	13	3	7	10	5	7	11	4	21	2	199
Potato S	16	8	10	17	11	9	13	1	10	6	10	9	3	4	4	3	11		>144
Potato X	24	29	17	19	18	13	46	3	14	8	12	10	2	12	12	2	10	6	257
Potato Y	~20	15	9	22	10	~11	15	1	13	10	10	11	7	5	11	5	12	2	190
Potato yellow dwarf†	10.3	5.6	7.1	9.4	4.8	3.9	3.3	ND	4.1	2.8	5.2	8.6	2.7	2.1	6.0	1.0	3.6		(33 × 10³)
	20.0	15.6	16.4	20.0	10.2	17.4	21.0	ND	7.2	5.8	12.6	14.0	5.8	6.2	9.8	1.0	7.8		(56 × 10³)
	13.6	9.4	12.8	6.0	5.7	6.1	5.1	ND	4.6	1.2	7.9	6.8	3.5	3.0	2.3	1.0	3.9		(78 × 10³)

	11.2	7.2	5.0	7.9	11.4	5.9	5.1	2.0	9.7	1.8	3.7	7.2	1.9	3.5	4.1	2.7	7.6	2.0	
Prunus necrotic ringspot‡																				
Southern bean mosaic	18	32	26	18	14	19	24	3	21	7	12	28	10	4	7	2	20	5	270
Sowbane mosaic	16	13	14	12	12	16	15	2	13	5	9	12	7	4	12	3	8	3	176
Squash mosaic	21	17	16	14	10	15	19		9	4	14	19	10	3	8	3	7		>189
Tobacco etch	25	13	9	23	8	13	19	1	12	10	5	13	7	5	10	6	13	2	194
Tobacco rattle	20	10	21	16	13	7	21		8	3	3	14	5	11	15	1	10		>178
Tobacco ringspot	17	13	14	14	11	15	15		11	3	11	14	6	10	9	6	8		>177
Tomato bushy stunt (average of two proteins)																			
strain BS-3	43	43	35	22	16	41	36	4	44	3	15	44	10	14	14	5	19		>408
strain BS-9	43	43	32	23	16	42	30		33	3	12	46	11	12	13	4	20		>383
Tomato ringspot	16	15	16	18	12	18	15	5	10	3	13	24	7	15	10	5	11	5	218
Tulare apple mosaic§	9.5	6.0	9.5	6.6	10.8	7.6	9.4	0.6	8.2	1.7	2.2	3.2	3.7	5.5	6.4	1.1	4.1	4.0	
Turnip crinkle§																			
a	9.7	6.5	8.7	13.0	4.1	7.8	5.9	1	6.0	1.5	4.1	7.2	4.8	5.9	7.2	1.6	6.0	4	(28 × 10³)
b	9.6	9.0	6.7	14.7	4.0	5.3	7.6		7.2	1.9	3.5	9.0	3.9	4.9	7.0	1.0	4.8		(40 × 10³)
c	8.6	5.4	8.0	15.0	3.8	10.1	5.6		5.0	0	3.5	6.7	3.1	3.7	13.3	1.5	7.5		(~80 × 10³)
Turnip mosaic	29	16	10	23	9	15	17	1	12	11	10	20	8	9	13	8	17	3	231
Turnip yellow mosaic	11	26	16	15	20	8	15	4	14	4	15	18	3	5	7	3	3	2	189
White clover mosaic	12	11	10	9	8	7	19	2	7	2	9	10	3	6	8	2	6	2	133
Wild cucumber mosaic	15	13	26	11	19	9	16	2	12	1	13	24	3	8	9	3	5	1	190

* Excepting the tobacco mosaic family and tobacco necrosis and satellite viruses, which are given in Table 4.

† The two predominant coat proteins and the membrane protein; analyses per minimal molecular weight (1 His). To be multiplied by respectively 3.6, 2.8, and 7.8 to obtain residues per mole.

‡ Data given as mole percent.

§ Data given as gram-residue percent.

TABLE 3

Covirus, Satellite, and Multi-Nucleic Acid Virus Systems

Coviruses

Cowpea mosaic virus group	Two dissimilar isometric particles or their two different RNAs: Both needed for infection (information for essential gene, possibly replicase, distributed over both RNAs).
Tobacco rattle virus group	Two dissimilar rod-shaped particles, two different RNAs: The longer is alone infective but yields unstable virus (sterile lesions) (coat protein information in shorter RNA, longer RNA carrying all genes essential for infection and lesion formation).
Alfalfa mosaic virus group	Four dissimilar rod-shaped to isometric particles, four different RNAs: The three largest particles or all four RNAs needed for infection (coat protein information in the two shortest RNAs).
Brome mosaic virus group	Three very similar isometric particles, four different RNAs: The three particles or the three larger RNAs needed for infectivity (coat protein information in the two shortest RNAs).

Satellite and tobacco necrosis virus:

	Two unrelated particles and RNAs: Necrosis infectivity carried by large particle or RNA alone; satellite infectivity only by combination of both (the satellite believed to carry only its own protein information and to use the replicase and any other components needed for infection from the helper virus, tobacco necrosis).

Multi-nucleic acid viruses*:

Influenza virus, oncornaviruses, diplornaviruses	One particle contains several or many (3–13) RNA molecules (single- or double-stranded), which carry different bits of information.

Typical RNA viruses

	One particle containing one molecule of RNA.

* The only plant viruses in this group are the diplornaviruses, rice dwarf virus, and wound tumor virus.

TABLE 4

Amino Acid Composition of the Tobacco Mosaic Virus Family and the Tobacco Necrosis Viruses and Their Satellites

Class	Example	Asp	Thr	Ser	Glu	Pro	Gly	Ala	Cys	Val	Met	Ile	Leu	Tyr	Phe	Lys	His	Arg	Trp	Total	ΔA*
Tobacco mosaic viruses																					
A	Wild type	18	16	16	16	8	6	14	1	14	0	9	12	4	8	2	0	11	3	158	
B	Dahlemense	17	17	16	19	8	6	11	1	15	1	7	13	5	8	2	0	9	3	158	8
C	U2	22	19	10	16	10	5	17	1	12	2	8	11	6	8	1	0	8	2	158	16
D	HR	17	13	13	22	8	4	18	1	10	3	8	11	7	6	2	1	10	2	156	20
E	ORSV	20	21	12	15	9	7	11	1	10	3	8	14	7	7	1	0	9	3	158	17
F	Cucumber 3	17	12	22	10	8	5	18	0	14	0	5	13	4	10	3	0	9	1	151	18
G	Cucumber 4	18	12	23	10	9	5	20	0	14	0	7	12	4	11	4	0	10	1	160	17
H	CGMMV-C	20	10	24	10	6	9	21	0	7	0	7	18	4	9	4	2	8	2	161	30
I	CGMMV-W	18	12	21	10	10	5	18	0	13	0	8	12	4	12	4	0	10	1	158	16
Tobacco necrosis viruses																					
	AC36	27	24	21	30	23	12	20	3	21	9	17	15	17	18	18	1.5	21		>298	
	Urbana Isol.	34	19	21	24	23	25	41	5	18	5	20	21	15	10	10	1	20		313	
	Satellite																				
	SV1	31	19	14	17	4	18	16	1	14	5	14	16	4	7	8	4	14	2	208	
	SV2	25	26	17	18	3	12	18	2	19	3	13	9	4	11	8	3	15	1	207	
	SVₑ	27	25	12	18	4	8	9	2	13	4	13	20	6	11	11	6	24		>209	

* Net exchanges compared to Class A.

```
                                              *  ** 10*      *             20** **
Wild type:  AcSer-Tyr-Ser-Ile-Thr-Thr-Pro-Ser-Gln-Phe-Val-Phe-Leu-Ser-Ser-Ala-Trp-Ala-Asp-Pro-Ile-Glu-Leu-
Dahlemense:   "    "   "    "   "   "   "   Ser  "   "  Phe  "    "   "   "   "    "   "   "   "   "   "   "
U2:         Pro    "  Thr   "  Asn   "   "   "   "  Tyr  "   "  Ala-Tyr  "   "   "  Val  "
HR:         AcSer  "  Asn   "  Thr-Asn-Ser-Asn  "  Tyr-Gln  " Phe-Ala-Ala-Val-Trp  " Glu  "  Thr-Pro-Met-

             *  **                         30**
Wild type:  Ile-Asn-Leu- Cys-Thr-Asn-Ala-Leu-Gly-Asn-Gln-Phe-Gln-Thr-Gln-Gln-Ala-Arg-Thr-Val-Val-Gln-Arg  40
Dahlemense: Leu  "  Val   "   "   "   "   "   "   Ser-Ser  "   "   "   "   "   "   "   "  Thr  "  Gln
U2:         Ile  "  Leu   "   " Asn-Ala  "   "   "   "   "   "   "   "   "   "   "   "   "   "   "
HR:         Leu  "  Gln   " Val-Ser  "   "  Ser Gln-Ser-Tyr  "   "   "  Ala-Gly  " Asp  " Arg  "

             50          *   **  ***            60  *      **   ***       *
Wild type:  Gln-Phe-Ser-Gln-Val-Trp-Lys-Pro-Ser-Pro-Gln-Val-Thr-Val-Arg-Phe-Pro-Asp-Ser-Asp-Phe-Lys-Val-
Dahlemense:  "   "  Ser-Glu-Val  "   "   "  Phe  "  Gln-Ser  "   "   "   "  Gly-Asp-Val-Tyr-Lys
U2:          "   "  Ala-Asp-Ala  "   "   "  Ser  "  Val-Met  "   "   "  Ala-Ser-Asp-Phe-Tyr  "
HR:          "   "   " Asn-Leu-Leu-Ser-Thr-Ile-Val-Ala-Pro-Asn-Gln  "   "   "  Asp-Thr-Gly-Phe-Arg  "

CGMM-W:                                                                                            Asn-Arg-
CGMM-C:
             70       **                        80  **                         90
Wild type:  Tyr-Arg-Tyr-Asn-Ala-Val-Leu-Asp-Pro-Leu-Val-Thr-Ala-Leu-Leu-Gly-Ala-Phe-Asp-Thr-Arg
Dahlemense:  "   "   "   "  Ala-Val  "   "   "   "  Ile  "   "   "   "   "  Gly-Thr  "   "   "
U2:          "   "  Ser-Thr  "   "   "   "   "   "  Asn-Ser  "   "   "
HR:          "  Val-Asn-Ser-Ala-Val-Ile-Lys  "   "  Tyr-Glu  "   "  Met-Lys-Ser  "
```

```
                                                    100                            *
CGMM-W:     Val-Ile-Glu-Val-Val-Asp-Pro-Ser-Asn-Pro-Thr-Thr-Ala-Glu-Ser-Leu-Asn-Ala-Val-Lys-Arg-Thr-Asp-
CGMM-C:     Ala  "   "   "   "  Glx-Asx  "  Asp  "  Ser  "  Gly  "  Ala  "   Thr  "  Asp  "

                        *                                            **
Wild type:  Ile  "   "  Glu-Asn-Gln-Ala-Asn  "  Thr  "  Ala  "  Thr  "  Asp  "  Arg  "  Val  "
Dahlemense:  "   "   "   "   "  Gln-Ser  "   "   "   "   "   "   "   "   "   "   "
U2:          "  Glx  "  Asx-Asx-Glx-Ala-Asx  "   "   "  Val(Thr,Pro,Asn,Ile)Glx-Glx
HR:          "  Gln-Thr-Glu-Glu-Gln-Ser-Arg  "  Ser-Ala-Ser-Gln-Val-Ala-Asn-Ala-Thr-Gln
```

```
                    120
CGMM-W:     Asp-Ala-Ser-Thr-Ala-Ala-Arg
CGMM-C:      "   "   "   "   "   "  His
```

```
                               *          **  130                 **       *         **
Wild type:  Thr-Val  " Ile-Arg-Ser-Ala-Ile-Asn-Asn-Leu-Ile-Val-Glu-Leu-Ile-Arg-Gly-Thr-Gly-Ser-
Dahlemense:  "   "    "   "   "   "   "   "   "   "  Val-Asn  "   "   "   "  Val  "   "   "  Leu-
U2:          "   "    "   "   "   "  Ala-Ser  "   "   "  Ala  "   "   "   "   "   "   "  Met-
HR:         Ser-Gln  "  Ser-Gln  "  Gln-Leu  "  Leu  "  Ser-Asn-His-Gly  "  Tyr-
```

```
            *  140*                   *     *  150                 **
Wild type:  Tyr-Asn-Arg-Ser-Ser-Phe-Glu-Ser-Ser-Ser-Gly-Leu-Val-Trp-Thr-Ser-Gly-Pro-Ala-Thr-
Dahlemense: Tyr  " Gln-Asn-Thr  " Ser-Met  "   "   "   "   "   "   "   "  Ala  " Ser
U2:         Phe  " Gln-Ala-Gly  " Thr-Ala  "   "   "   "   "   "   "  Thr-Thr  " Thr
HR:         Met  " Arg  " Glu  " Ala-Ile  "   "  Pro  "   "   "   "   "  Ala  "   "
```

Fig. 1. The amino acid sequence of the coat proteins of TMV strains. The wild type, Dahlemense, U2, and HR strains are representatives of classes A, B, C, and D. CGMM viruses, partially sequenced, are cucumber green mottle mosaic virus strains (strains W and C). Asterisks indicate amino acids which have been found to be replaced by others once (*) or more frequently (**) in chemically produced mutant (usually only one, two, or quite rarely three replacements in one mutant).

AcMet–Glu–Ile–Asp–Lys–Glu–Leu–Ala–Pro–Gln–Asp–Arg–Thr–Val–Thr–Val–
Ala–Thr–Val–Leu–Pro–Ala–Val–Pro–Gly–Pro–Ser–Pro–Leu–Thr–Ile–Lys–
Gln–Pro–Phe–Gln–Ser–Glu–Val–Leu–Phe–Ala–Gly–Thr–Lys–Asp–Ala–Glu–
Ala–Ser–Leu–Thr–Ile–Ala–Asn–Ile–Asp–Ser–Val–Ser–Thr–Leu–Thr–Thr–
Phe–Tyr–Arg–His–Ala–Ser–Leu–Glu–Ser–Leu–Trp–Val–Thr–Ile–His–Pro–
Thr–Leu–Gln–Ala–Pro–Thr–Phe–Pro–Thr–Thr–Val–Gly–Val–Cys–Trp–Val–
Pro–Ala–Asn–Ser–Pro–Val–Thr–Pro–Ala–Gln–Ile–Thr–Lys–Thr–Tyr–Gly–
Gly–Gln–Ile–Phe–Cys–Ile–Gly–Gly–Ala–Ile–Asn–Thr–Leu–Ser–Pro–Leu–
Ile–Val–Lys–Cys–Pro–Leu–Glu–Met–Met–Asn–Pro–Arg–Val–Lys–Asp–Ser–
Ile–Gln–Tyr–Leu–Asp–Ser–Pro–Lys–Leu–Leu–Ile–Ser–Ile–Thr–Ala–Gln–
Pro–Thr–Ala–Pro–Pro–Ala–Ser–Thr–Cys–Ile–Ile–Thr–Val–Ser–Gly–Thr–
Leu–Ser–Met–His–Ser–Pro–Leu–Ile–Thr–Asp–Thr–Ser–Thr–COOH

Fig. 2.   The amino acid sequence of the turnip yellows mosaic virus (Peter *et al.*, 1972).

References (Section B)

Aapola, A. I. E., and Rochow, W. F., 1971, *Virology* **46**, 127.

Agrawal, H. O., 1967, *J. Ultrastruct. Res.* **17**, 84.

Atabekov, J. G., Novikov, V. K., Kiselev, N. A., Kaftanova, A. S., and Egorov, A. M., 1968, *Virology* **36**, 620.

Bancroft, J. B., 1971, *Virology* **45**, 830.

Bancroft, J. B., and Flack, I. H., 1972, *J. Gen. Virol.* **15**, 247.

Barnett, O. W., and Fulton, R. W., 1969, *Virology* **39**, 556.

Barnett, O. W., Zoeten, G. A. de, and Gaard, G., 1971, *Phytopathology* **61**, 926.

Bercks, R., Huth, W., Koenig, R., Lesemann, D., Paul, H. L., and Quarfurth, G., 1971, *Phytopathol. Z.* **71**, 341.

Biddle, P. G., and Tinsley, T. W., 1971, *New Phytol.* **70**, 61.

Bol, J. F., and Van Vloten-Doting, L., 1973, *Virology* **51**, 102.

Bond, W. P., and Pirone, T. P., 1971, *Phytopathol. Z.* **71**, 56.

Brakke, M. V., and Van Pelt, N., 1970, *Virology* **42**, 699.

Brandes, J., and Bercks, R., 1965, *Adv. Virus Res.* **11**, 1.

Brandes, J., and Luisoni, E., 1966, *Phytopathol. Z.* **57**, 277.

Brunt, A. A., 1966a, *Ann. Appl. Biol.* **58**, 13.

Brunt, A. A., 1966b, *Virology* **28**, 778.

Brunt, A. A., and Kenten, R. H., 1971, *Ann. Appl. Biol.* **69**, 235.

Brunt, A. A., and Kitagima, E. W., 1973, *Phytopathol. Z.* **76**, 265.

Butler, P. J. G., 1970, *J. Molec. Biol.* **52**, 589.

Chen, M. -J., and Shikata, E., 1971, *Virology* **46**, 786.

Chessin, M., Zaitlin, M., and Solberg, R. A., 1967, *Phytopathology* **57**, 452.

Civerolo, E. L., Semancik, J. S., and Weathers, L. G., 1968, *Phytopathology* **58**, 1481.

Cohn, E., Tanne, E., and Nitzany, F. E., 1970, *Phytopathology* **60**, 181.

Converse, R. H., and Lister, R. M., 1969, *Phytopathology* **59**, 325.

Cooper, J. I., and Mayo, M. A., 1972, *J. Gen. Virol.* **16**, 285.

Damirdagh, I. S., and Shepherd, R. J., 1970, *Virology* **40**, 84.

de Sequeira, O. A., and Lister, R. M., 1969, *Phytopathology* **59**, 1740.

Dieleman-van Zaayen, A., 1972, *Virology* **47**, 94.

Diener, T. O., 1972, *Virology* **50**, 606.

Diener, T. O., and Lawson, R. H., 1973, *Virology* **51**, 94.

Duffus, J. E., 1969, *Phytopathology* **59**, 1668.

Duffus, J. E., 1973, *Adv. Virus Res.* **18**, in press.

Duffus, J. E., and Russell, G. E., 1972, *Phytopathology* **62**, 1274.

Francki, R. I. B., and Grivell, C. J., 1970, *Virology* **42**, 969.

Francki, R. I. B., and Grivell, C. J., 1972, *Virology* **48**, 305.

Freitag, J. H., and Milne, K. S., 1970, *Phytopathology* **60**, 166.

Fujisawa, I., Rubio-Huertos, M., and Matsui, M., 1971, *Phytopathology* **61**, 681.

Fulton, R. W., 1967, *Phytopathology* **57**, 1197.

Fulton, R. W., 1968, *Phytopathology* **58**, 635.

Gálvez, G. E., 1968, *Virology* **35**, 418.

Geelen, J. L. M. C., Van Kammen, A., and Verduin, B. J. M., 1972, *Virology* **49**, 205.

Ghabrial, S. A., Shepherd, R. J., and Grogan, R. G., 1967, *Virology* **33**, 17.

Gibbs, A. J., Hecht-Poinar, E., Woods, R. D., and McKee, R. K., 1966, *J. Gen. Microbiol.* **44**, 177.

Gibbs, A. J., Girssani-Bells, G., and Smith, H. G., 1968, *Ann. Appl. Biol.* **61**, 99.

Gonsalves, D., and Shepherd, R. J., 1972, *Virology* **48**, 709.

Gumpf, D. J., 1971, *Virology* **43**, 588.

Hariharasubramanian, V., and Siegel, A., 1969, *Virology* **37**, 203.

Herold, F., and Munz, K., 1967, *J. Gen. Virol.* **1**, 227.

Hiebert, E., 1970, *Phytopathology* **60**, 1295.

Hiebert, E., Purcifull, D. E., Christie, R. G., and Christie, S. R., 1971, *Virology* **43**, 638.

Hill, J. H., and Shepherd, R. J., 1972a, *Virology* **47**, 807.

Hill, J. H., and Shepherd, R. J., 1972b, *Virology* **47**, 817.

Hoeffert, L. L., Esau, K., and Duffus, J. E., 1970, *Virology* **42**, 814.

Hull, R., 1972, *J. Gen. Virol.* **17**, 111.

Hull, R., and Lane, L. C., 1973, *Virology* **55**, 1.

Huth, W., 1968, *Phytopathol. Z.* **62**, 300.

Jackson, A. O., and Brakke, M. K., 1973, *Virology* **55**, 483.

Jones, A. T., Kinninmonth, A. M., and Roberts, I. M., 1973, *J. Gen. Virol.* **18**, 61.

Kado, C. I., and Black, D. R., 1968, *Virology* **36**, 137.

Kalmakoff, J., and Tremaine, J. H., 1967, *Virology* **33**, 10.

Kaper, J. M., and Waterworth, H. E., 1973, *Virology* **51**, 183.

Kaper, J. M., and Wirt, C. K., 1972, *Prep. Biochem.* **2**(3), 251.

Kassanis, B., Woods, R. D., and White, R. F., 1972, *J. Gen. Virol.* **14**, 123.

Kenten, R. H., and Legg, J. T., 1967, *J. Gen. Virol.* **1**, 465.

Lane, L. C., and Kaesberg, P., 1971, *Nature New Biol.* **232**, 40.

Lastra, R., and Munz, K., 1969, *Phytopathology* **59**, 1429.

Lauffer, M. A., and Stevens, C. L., 1968, *Adv. Virus Res.* **13**, 1.

Lawson, R. H., and Hearon, S., 1970, *Virology* **41**, 30.

Lee, P. E., 1968, *Virology* **34**, 583.

Lesemann, D., 1972, *J. Gen. Virol.* **16**, 273.

Lewandowski, L. J., and Traynor, B. L., 1972, *J. Virol.* **10**, 1053.

Lin, M. T., and Campbell, R. N., 1972, *Virology* **48**, 30.

Lister, R. M., and Bancroft, J. B., 1970, *Phytopathology* **60**, 689.

Lister, R. M., and Hadidi, A. F., 1971, *Virology* **45**, 240.

Luisoni, E., Lovisolo, D., Kitagawa, Y., and Shikata, E., 1973, *Virology* **52**, 281.

Martelli, G. P., and Russo, M., 1972, *J. Gen. Virol.* **15**, 193.

Matthews, R. E. F., and Ralph, R. K., 1966, *Adv. Virus Res.* **12**, 273.

Mayo, M. A., and Jones, A. T., 1973, *J. Gen. Virol.* **19**, 245.

Miki, T., and Oshima, N., 1972a, *Virology* **48**, 386.

Miki, T., and Oshima, N., 1972b, *J. Gen. Virol.* **15**, 179.

Milne, K. S., and Grogan, R. G., 1969, *Phytopathology* **59**, 809.

Mink, G. T., 1969, *Phytopathology* **59**, 1889.

Minson, A. C., and Darby, G., 1973, *J. Gen. Virol.* **19**, 253.

Miura, K. -I., Kimura, I., and Suzuki, N., 1966, *Virology* **28**, 571.

Moline, H. E., McDaniel, G. L., and Mayhew, D. E., 1971, *Phytopathology* **61**, 903.

Moore, B. J., and Scott, H. A., 1971, *Phytopathology* **61**, 831.

Mundry, K. W., and Priess, H., 1971, *Virology* **46**, 86.

Murant, A. F., and Roberts, I. M., 1971, *J. Gen. Virol.* **10**, 65.

Murant, A. F., Goold, R. A., Roberts, I. M., and Cathro, J., 1969, *J. Gen. Virol.* **4**, 329.

Murant, A. F., Mayo, M. A., Harrison, B. D., and Goold, R. A., 1972, *J. Gen. Virol.* **16**, 327.

Murant, A. F., Mayo, M. A., Harrison, B. D., and Goold, R. A., 1973, *J. Gen. Virol.* **19**, 275.

Nozu, Y., Tochihara, H., Komuro, Y., and Okada, Y., 1971, *Virology* **45**, 577.

Paul, H. L., 1962, *Phytopathol. Z.* **43**, 315.

Peter, R., Stehelin, D., Reinbolt, J., Collot, D., and Duranton, H., 1972, *Virology* **49**, 615.

Peters, D., and Kitajima, E. W., 1970, *Virology* **41**, 135.

Peters, D., and van Loon, L. C., 1968, *Virology* **35**, 597.

Plumb, R. T., and Vince, D. A., 1971, *J. Gen. Virol.* **13**, 357.

Price, W. C., 1966, *Virology* **29**, 285.

Randles, J. W., and Francki, R. I. B., 1972, *Virology* **50**, 297.

Reeder, G. S., Knudson, D. L., and MacLeod, R., 1972, *Virology* **50**, 301.

Rees, M. W., and Short, M. N., 1965, *Virology* **26**, 596.

Rees, M. W., Short, M. N., and Kassanis, B., 1970, *Virology* **40**, 448.

Rochow, W. F., Aapola, A. I. E., Brakke, M. K., and Carmichael, L. E., 1971, *Virology* **46**, 117.

Ross, J. P., 1969, *Phytopathology* **59**, 829.

Ross, J. P., 1970, *Phytopathology* **60**, 1798.

Russell, G. J., Follett, E. A. C., Subak-Sharpe, J. H., and Harrison, B. D., 1971, *J. Gen. Virol.* **11**, 129.

Russo, M., and Martelli, G. P., 1973, *Virology* **52**, 39.

Sänger, H. L., 1969, *J. Virol.* **3**, 304.

Schmelzer, K., 1967, *Phytopathol. Z.* **58**, 59.

Scott, H. A., and Moore, B. J., 1972, *Virology* **50**, 613.

Semancik, J. S., and Weathers, L. G., 1972, *Virology* **49**, 622.

Serjeant, P., 1967, *Ann. Appl. Biol.* **59**, 31.

Shepherd, R. J., Fulton, J. P., and Wakeman, R. J., 1969, *Phytopathology* **59**, 219.

Shepherd, R. J., Bruening, G. E., and Wakeman, R. J., 1970, *Virology* **41**, 339.

Siegel, A., and Wildman, S. G., 1954, *Phytopathology* **44**, 277.

Snazelle, T. E., Bancroft, J. B., and Ullstrup, A. J., 1971, *Phytopathology* **61**, 1059.

Stace-Smith, R., and Tremaine, J. H., 1973, *Virology* **51**, 401.

Stace-Smith, R., Reichmann, M. E., and Wright, N. S., 1965, *Virology* **25**, 487.

Sun, M. K. C., and Hebert, T. T., 1971, *Phytopathology* **61**, 914.

Symons, R. H., Rees, M. W., Short, M. N., and Markham, R., 1963, *J. Molec. Biol.* **6**, 1.

Taylor, R. H., Smith, P. R., Reinganum, C., and Gibbs, A. J., 1968, *Austral. J. Biol. Sci.* **21**, 929.

Tomlinson, J. A., 1964, *Ann. Appl. Biol.* **53**, 95.

Tremaine, J. H., 1970, *Virology* **42**, 611.

Tremaine, J. H., 1972, *Virology* **48,** 582.

Tremaine, J. H., and Stace-Smith, R., 1968, *Virology* **35,** 102.

Tung, J. -S., and Knight, C. A., 1972a, *Virology* **48,** 574.

Tung, J. -S., and Knight, C. A., 1972b, *Virology* **49,** 214.

van Regenmortel, M. H. V., Hendry, D. A., and Baltz, T., 1972, *Virology* **49,** 647.

Varma, A., Gibbs, A. J., Woods, R. D., and Finch, J. T., 1968, *J. Gen. Virol.* **2,** 107.

Wang, A. L., and Knight, C. A., 1967, *Virology* **31,** 101.

Waterworth, H. E., and Kaper, J. M., 1972, *Phytopathology* **62,** 959.

Weintraub, M., and Ragetli, H. W. J., 1970, *Virology* **40,** 868.

Wetter, C., 1960, *Arch. Mikrobiol.* **37,** 278.

Wetter, C., Quantz, L., and Brandes, J., 1962, *Phytopathol. Z.* **43,** 151.

Wilson, H. R., Tollin, P., and Rahman, A., 1973, *J. Gen. Virol.* **18,** 181.

Wu, G. -J., and Bruening, G., 1971, *Virology* **46,** 596.

Zaumeyer, W. J., and Goth, R. W., 1964, *Phytopathology* **54,** 1378.

Section C

Viruses of Protists

The viruses of protists, mostly of bacteria, will be listed alphabetically, Roman letters being followed by the corresponding Greek letters, followed by arabic numbers, followed by Roman numbers. The letter ϕ at the beginning of such symbols (presumably standing for phage, and not consistently used for the same phages) will be omitted throughout: thus ϕX174 is X 174.

Frequently phages are not named at all, but only described in general terms as infecting certain protists. We will list such hosts and their anonymous viruses alphabetically at the end. Many phages of *Escherichia coli* also attack other related bacterial species and vice versa. Thus the assignments to *Escherichia coli, Salmonella typhimurium, Bacillus subtilis, Alcaligenes faecalis,* etc. may be arbitrary.

Since most viruses of protists contain double-stranded DNA, this is its state unless otherwise specified (e.g., single-stranded DNA, single- or double-stranded RNA, or unknown nucleic acid). Many phages are described only in terms of their nucleic acid and often only their base composition, as derived from their buoyant density in CsCl or more rarely their T_m. As in Sections A and B of this catalogue, we will give data on the particle first, followed by nucleic acid data, protein data, and particular biological data. Unless otherwise specified, phages are virulent and lyse the host cell. One or two recent references will be given when available to facilitate the reader's search for further information.

A (*Escherichia coli*). Isometric virus containing single-stranded circular DNA, serologically related to X 174. (Taketo and Kuno, 1969.)

Ac (*Salmonella typhimurium*). Typical phage with DNA of 43% (G+C).

121

Ac 20 (*Asticacaulis*). Phage with hexagonal head and simple tail.

AE 2 (*Escherichia coli*). Filamentous particles of 5 × 800 nm, 43 S, containing 14% single-stranded DNA. A/G/T/C = 26/21/32/21. (Panter and Symons, 1966.)

AfVF, AfVS (*Aspergillus foetidus*). Isometric 40 nm particles, heterodisperse in density and containing two electrophoretic classes. Both contain several species of double-stranded RNA; the faster (F) contains RNA of molecular weights 2.31, 1.87, 1.70, and 1.44 × 10^6; the slower (S) RNA of molecular weights 2.76 and 2.24 × 10^6. These various RNAs are separately encapsidated to give particles of different buoyant densities. Such viruses may account for the interferon activity of these fungi. (Banks *et al.*, 1970; Ratti and Buck, 1972.)

AS-1 (*Anacystis nidulans* and *Synechococcus cedrorum*, unicellular species of blue-green algae). (The viruses are serologically unrelated to other known viruses of blue-green algae). Polyhedral 90 nm diameter head with 22.5 × 244 nm tail. The tail contracts to 93 nm, revealing an 8 nm core; the base plate is 40 nm across with short pins and fibers. The 260/280 nm absorbance ratio is 1.88. The virus contains DNA of about 54% (G+C). The virus has an 8.5 hour latent period, a 7.5 hour rise period, and a burst size of 50 PFU per infected cell. (Safferman *et al.*, 1972.)

AT 298 (*Streptococcus*). Temperate transducing phage. (Colón *et al.*, 1971.)

A 5/A 6 (*Alcaligenes faecalis*). Related to A 25. (Maré *et al.*, 1966.)

A 11/A 79 (*Alcaligenes faecalis*). Phage with contractile tail but no appendages. (Maré *et al.*, 1966.)

A 11 (*Azotobacter vinelandii*) (A 11 to A 14 are serologically interrelated). Particles with 120 nm head diameter, 20 × 180 nm contractile tail, and DNA of 53% (G+C). (Knovicka *et al.*, 1972.)

A 12 (*Azotobacter*). Isometric particles of 56 nm diameter with particle weight 76 × 10^6, short noncontractile tail, 58% DNA (44 × 10^6 mol. wt.), 58% (G+C). (Domingo *et al.*, 1972.)

A 13 (*Azotobacter*). Particle of 60 nm head diameter, 10 × 170 nm concontractile tail. The DNA contains 52% (G+C). (Knovicka *et al.*, 1972.)

A 14 (*Azotobacter*). Particles of 470 × 10^6 daltons, with 120 nm head diameter, 20×180 nm contractile tail, and 34% DNA of 165×10^6 mol. wt. and 53% (G+C). (Knovicka *et al.*, 1972.)

A 20 (*Asticacaulis*). Typical phage with long noncontractile tail with appendages.

A 21, A 22, A 23, A 24 (*Azotobacter vinelandii*) (serologically interrelated phages). Isometric particles of 57 nm diameter with short noncontractile tail, 78×10^6 dalton particle weight; the DNA (58%) of molecular weight 44×10^6 is 57% (G+C). (Domingo *et al.*, 1972; Knovicka *et al.*, 1972.)

A 25 (*Streptococcus*) (related to GT 234). Hexagonal head of 47 nm diameter and long noncontractile tail (8×185 nm) with terminal knob. Virulent transducing phage. (Colón *et al.*, 1971.)

A 31 (*Azotobacter vinelandii*). Isometric particles of 61 nm diameter with long noncontractile tail, 175×10^6 dalton particle weight, 26% DNA of 52% (G+C) (uncertain, 69% by T_m). (Domingo *et al.*, 1972.)

A 41 (*Azotobacter vinelandii*). Unstable particles with short noncontractile tail. DNA of 46×10^6 mol. wt.

A 64/A 62 (*Alcaligenes faecalis*). Hexagonal particles with long, thin tails; 61% (G+C) (Maré *et al.*, 1966.)

A 422 (*Brucella* spp.). Identical to Tbilisi phage.

α (*Salmonella* spp.) 55% (G+C).

α (*Bacillus tiberius* or *B. megaterium*). Temperate icosahedral phage of 400 S containing 33×10^6 mol. wt. DNA (40 S) of 41% (G+C), with an average of one interruption per chain. This was the first DNA virus in which it was found possible to separate the strands by density gradients (1.717 and 1.724 g/ml in CsCl). (Cordes *et al.*, 1961; Strniste and Taylor, 1972.)

α 15, 17 (*Escherichia coli*). Probably members of group IV of RNA phages; *see* ZG (A/U = 1.02) (related to f 2?).

B, BL (*Corynebacterium diphtheriae*). Phage with long noncontractile tail. (Mathews *et al.*, 1966.)

BF (*Escherichia coli*) (related to T 5). (Shinozawa, 1973.)

BM (*Bacillus megaterium*). Particles of 60 nm diameter with 15×130 nm tail.

BO 1, BO 2a, BO 2b (*Mycobacterium smegmatis* and *M. phlei*). Hexagonal heads (BO 1 elongated) and long noncontractile tails, DNA of 71 or 72% (G+C). (Kraiss *et al.*, 1973.)

B 1 (*Pseudomonas aeruginosa*). Phage with long noncontractile tail. (Takeya and Amako, 1966).

B 179 (*Agrobacterium radiobacter*).

β (*Corynebacterium diphtheriae*). Particles of 55 × 61 nm head, 10 × 287 nm tail. (Nagington and Carne, 1971.)

β (*Escherichia coli*). Member of group I of RNA phages (*see* f 2).

β 22 (*Bacillus subtilis*). Large virulent phage unrelated to SP 82. 100 nm diameter head and 300-nm-long tail.

C (*Nocardia erythropolis*). Typical particles of 52 nm diameter with 10 × 192 nm tails. (Brownell and Adams, 1967.)

CbK (*Caulobacter crescentus*). Bacilliform particle, 62 × 210 nm, icosahedral, with flexible noncontractile tail of 290 nm. The linear DNA (57%) is 65% (G+C). (Leonard *et al.*, 1972.)

Cb 5 (*Caulobacter crescentus*). Isometric RNA phage, of 23 nm diameter, 71 S. It is extremely salt sensitive. The RNA is 31 S, A/G/U/C = 29/29/23/24. The protein contains histidine but is otherwise similar to coliphages. (Bendis and Shapiro, 1970.)

Cb8r (*Caulobacter*). Isometric RNA phage.

Cb 13 (*Caulobacter*). Phage with long bacilliform head and short tail.

Chi, *see* χ.

CP 1 (*Bacillus cereus*). Typical virulent phage; head 90 nm diameter; tail 20 × 160 nm; contains 56.7% DNA.

CP 3 (*Bacillus cereus*). Particles of 66 nm diameter; tail 12.5 × 276 nm; contains 51.9% DNA.

CP 51 (*Bacillus cereus*). Transducing phage with 90 nm diameter head, 20 × 160 nm tail, and 102 × 10⁶ particle weight. Contains DNA of 58 × 10⁶ mol. wt., 43% (G+C), and containing 5-hydroxymethyluracil instead of thymine. (Yelton and Thorne, 1971.)

CP 53 (*Bacillus cereus*). Transducing and lysogenizing phage. Head of 66 nm diameter, 13 × 276 nm tail, 29 × 10⁶ particle weight.

Contains 52% DNA of 17 × 10⁶ daltons, 37% (G+C) (and no unusual bases). (Yelton and Thorne, 1971.)

CT 1 (*Clostridium tetani*) (defective phage). Contains 32% (G+C).

CT 1–6 (*Rhizobium trifolii*). Isometric phages with contractile tails, containing DNA. CT 1, particles of 60 nm diameter, with 23 × 118 nm tails; CT 3, of 110 nm diameter, with 25 × 150 nm tails; CT 4, of 60 nm diameter, with 23 × 107 nm tails; CT 5, of 54 nm diameter, with 19 × 100 nm tails; CT 6, of 88 nm diameter, with 26 × 130 nm tails. (Barnet, 1972.)

C 1 (*Escherichia coli*). Large octahedral head (90 nm) and non-contractile sheath with pointed tip.

C 16 (*Escherichia coli*). Contains DNA of 34% (G+C).

C 21 (*Escherichia coli*). Only attacks K12 strains lacking galactose in cell wall.

C 31 (*Streptomyces coelicolor*). Temperate phage.

D (*Escherichia coli*). Temperate phage related to 186. (Lomovskaya *et al.*, 1972.)

DDII (*Shigella dysenteriae*). Icosahedral head of 55 nm diameter and short tail (15 × 20 nm), 480 S, particle weight 61 × 10⁶. The buoyant density in CsCl is 1.52 g/ml. The phage contains 47% DNA, 45% protein, 5% lipid. The DNA is linear (33 S), 30 × 10⁶ mol. wt., and 53% (G+C). (Nikolskaya *et al.*, 1972.)

DDVI (*Shigella dysenteriae*; also *Escherichia coli*). Elongated head (86 × 115 nm), and long contractile tail (18 × 130 nm); 895 S; buoyant density in CsCl 1.48 g/ml; 286 × 10⁶ daltons. The phage contains 48% linear DNA of 66 S, 143 × 10⁶ mol. wt., 65% (A+T), and containing glycosylated 5-hydroxymethylcytosine instead of cytosine. (Nikolskaya *et al.*, 1972.)

DDVII (*Shigella dysenteriae*; also *Escherichia coli*). Icosahedral head of 50 nm diameter and long noncontractile tail (4 × 135 nm); 530 S; 94 × 10⁶ in particle weight; buoyant density in CsCl 1.52 g/ml. The DNA of 41 S, 46 × 10⁶ mol. wt., is 45% (G+C). It seems to contain an unusual cationic sugar. (Nikolskaya *et al.*, 1972.)

D4, D29, D29a, D32 (*Mycobacterium* spp.).

D 6 (*Salmonella oranienburg*).

D 12 (*Escherichia coli*). Close relative of T-even phages.

D 108 (*Escherichia coli*). General transducing phage. Particles of 65 nm diameter with contractile tails of 22 × 137 nm. (Mise, 1971.)

δA (*Escherichia coli*). Filamentous 6 × 830 nm particle ($17 × 10^6$ in particle weight), containing 10% single-stranded DNA of $1.7 × 10^6$ mol. wt. (46 S). Density 1.30 g/ml. A/G/T/C = 26/21/33/20. (Nishihara and Watanabe, 1967.)

e (*Bacillus subtilis*). Contains DNA of 40% (G+C) with hydroxy-methyl-U instead of T. (Truffaut *et al.*, 1970.)

EC (*Nocardia erythropolis*). Typical particles of 52 nm diameter and 10 × 197 nm tails. (Brownell and Adams, 1967.)

EC9 (*Escherichia coli*). Filamentous phage with single-stranded DNA (*see* under Ff), 5 × 600 and 900 nm. Contains 15% DNA (39 S). A/G/T/C = 24/21/34/21.

EJ (*Escherichia coli*). Member of group II of RNA phages. (Miyake *et al.*, 1971.)

E1 (*Escherichia coli*). Octahedral head of 80 nm diameter, 100 nm contractile tail with cross-striations and four fibers but no well developed base plate.

ϵ^{15} (*Salmonella anatum*). Temperate phage. (Losick and Robbins, 1967.)

ϵ^{34} (*Salmonella* spp.). Can absorb only to cells lysogenic for ϵ^{15}.

η (*Serratia narcescens*). $73 × 10^6$ particle weight; buoyant density in CsCl is 1.495 g/ml. Contains about 45% DNA of $100 × 10^6$ mol. wt. The composition is 51% (A+T), part of the guanine being replaced by a not yet identified base of an absorbance maximum at all pHs above 280 nm. (Pons, 1966.)

F (*Bacillus subtilis*). Typical phage with DNA of 49% (G+C).

FA 5 (*Escherichia coli*). Member of group I of RNA phages (*see* f 2).

fca (*Escherichia coli*). Member of group I of RNA phages (*see* f 2).

fd (*Escherichia coli*). This phage represents the prototype for a considerable number of seemingly closely related filamentous phages (the Ff group, which also includes f 1, f 12, IKe, M 13, and ZJ 2), although some of these are of different lengths. The dimensions of the fd phage are 5.5 × 800 nm, the particle weight is said to be 11.3×10^3 (which is probably much too low), and the buoyant density is 1.30 g/ml in CsCl; 41 S. The helical pitch is probably 3.2 nm. The fine structure of these viruses is not yet known (see Electron micrograph XVII).

The phage contains a single molecule of single-stranded and circular DNA of molecular weight $1.7\text{-}2 \times 10^6$. The base composition of fd is $A/G/T/C = 24/20/36/20$.

The coat protein is unusually small (49 amino acids, mol. wt. 5158). The protein lacks cysteine, histidine, and arginine. The amino acid sequence of the fd coat protein is as follows:

Ala–Glu–Gly–Asp–Asp–Pro–Ala–Lys–Ala–Ala–Phe–Asp– (5, 10)

Ser–Leu–Gln–Ala–Ser–Ala–Thr–Glu–Tyr–Ile–Gly–Tyr– (15, 20)

Ala–Trp–Met–Val–Val–Val–Ile–Val–Gly–Ala–Thr–Ile– (25, 30, 35)

Gly–Ile–Lys–Leu–Phe–Lys–Lys–Phe–Thr–Ser–Lys–Ala–Ser (40, 45, 49)

The sequence shows three distinct regions, being predominantly hydrophilic in the N-terminal 20 residues, predominantly hydrophobic in the next 20 residues, and very basic in the C-terminal segment. About 1900 molecules make up a typical fd particle. The coat protein of ZJ 2 differs from this by only one amino acid replacement (Thr 35 → Ala) and one additional alanine (after Trp 26).

There also exist in these phage particles one or a very few molecules of a maturation protein, located probably at only one tip of the fibrous particle, of molecular weight 70,000.

These viruses infect by attaching themselves to the tip of pili, unlike the RNA phages, which attach themselves to their side. Since fd and most of the filamentous phages require F-pili they are male specific. The question whether these phages enter, or are drawn, *in toto* into the host cell, or whether they only "inject" their DNA, remains in dispute, but they certainly leave the host cell without causing lysis. (Marvin and Hoffman-Berling, 1963; Marvin and Hohn, 1969.)

F_F (*Escherichia coli*). Group of filamentous DNA phages adsorbing specifically to the tips of F-pili. (Members: f 1, fd, M 13, ZJ 12, Ec 9.) (Kay and Wakefield, 1972.)

FF 116 (*Pseudomonas* spp.). Generalized transducing phage, attaching to pili. Contains DNA of 39×10^6 daltons, 62% (G+C). (Pemberton, 1973.)

FI (*Escherichia coli*). Member of group IV of RNA phages, closely related to SP. (Miyake *et al.*, 1971.)

fr (*Escherichia coli*). Probably a member of group I of RNA phages, although not as closely related to f 2, the prototype, as are MS 2, R 17, and M 12.

The isometric particle has a diameter of about 21 nm (79 S) and 4.3×10^6 particle weight. It contains 29% RNA of about 1.2×10^6 mol. wt. (21 S), A/G/U/C = 24/27/24/25.

Detailed studies are available concerning the coat protein, which shows the same number of amino acids as f 2 (129) and sequence differences in only 23 locations, almost all of them representing exchanges of similar amino acids (hydrophilic for hydrophilic, hydrophobic for hydrophobic). The location of all prolines, cysteines, and most of the large side chain residues are the same (see Figure 4). (Marvin and Hoffmann-Berling, 1963; Wittmann-Liebold, 1966.)

F 1 (*Escherichia coli*). Large octahedral head and noncontractile sheath with forked tip.

f 1 (*Escherichia coli*). This filamentous phage is very similar if not identical to fd (*see* fd). For nucleotide sequence, see Figure 7.

f 2 (*Escherichia coli*). This is the first RNA-containing phage to be discovered. All RNA phages show considerable similarities, suggesting that they have common origins. On the other hand, at least four groups of *E. coli* RNA phages have been differentiated on the basis of serological differences or nonrelatedness. Group I contains f 2 and the very closely related phages MS 2, R 17, and M 12, as well as the less closely related phage fr. These four, which have been intensely studied, will be discussed together. Others, members of group I not yet studied and classified in detail, are phage 3, fca, FA 5, f 4, ZR, MY, GR, ZIK/1, ZJ 11. These, as apparently all RNA phages, infect by attaching themselves to the sides of bacterial F (= sex) pili, and are thus male-specific.

The phage f 2, as all RNA phages, is a typical picornavirus, an icosahedral particle of 23–25 nm diameter, lacking a tail or other surface features. The virion is of 80–82 S and has a particle weight of about 4×10^6.

These phages contain one molecule of singe-stranded RNA of about 1.2×10^6 mol. wt. and A/G/U/C ratios of 23/27/24/26. The A/U ratio of 0.94–0.98 is characteristic of group I, as contrasted to groups II and III (A/U = 0.85 and 0.79, respectively). The RNAs of all phages that were studied chemically (i.e., several of group I and Qβ) have 5′-terminal pppGpGpG- and 3′-terminal -CpCpCp-A. As far as the 3′-end is concerned, this is the same sequence found in most plant viral RNAs and seemingly related to the ability of the latter to simulate tRNAs and bind specific amino acids.

Over one-third of the nucleotide sequence of the RNA of MS 2 and smaller portions of the sequences for R 17 and f 2 have been established (see Figure 3). These appear to be identical for at least the first 140 nucleotides from the 5′-end, as well as for the 3′-terminal segment, but show isolated nucleotide replacements, usually of the last member of a codon, in coding parts of the RNA.

The coat protein of phage f 2 consists of 129 amino acids of known sequence (Figure 4), which differs from that of MS 2 and R 17 in only one amino acid replacement (Leu in position 88 → Met, and Glx → Lys, respectively), the latter two and M 12 apparently being the same. These proteins as well as all others of group I lack histidine.

The virions of these phages of group I and Qβ of group III also contain a single molecule of another protein, the A protein or maturation factor which plays critical roles in phage maturation and infection. The molecular weight of this protein is about 42,000, and its N-terminal sequence is (F-Met)-Arg-Ala-Phe-Ser-. Its last 45 amino acids have also recently been reported (see Figure 3). This protein contains five histidine residues.

To the extent that this was investigated, the RNA of all phages was found to serve directly as messenger, thus representing the positive strand, as is the case for all picornaviruses (of animals, plants, and bacteria) and the animal togaviruses (but not the other classes of RNA viruses). Besides coding for the coat protein and A protein discussed above, the RNA of these phages also codes for a peptide chain, which in conjunction with three host protein chains forms the RNA polymerase. The N-terminal sequence of the viral polypeptide chain is (F-Met)-Ser-Lys-Thr-Thr-Lys-. Its molecular weight is about 65,000 (Figure 3).

The order of the three genes has been shown to be 5′–A protein–coat protein–polymerase chain–3′, with noncoding segments at both ends and between the genes; one completely known intergenic sequence is 30 nucleotides long after the two termination codons following the last amino acid of the coat protein (of R 17 and MS 2); another between the A protein and coat protein gene is

26 nucleotides long (see Figure 3). (Contreras *et al.*, 1973; Fedoroff and Zinder, 1973.)

f 4 (*Escherichia coli*). Member of group I of RNA phages (*see* f 2).

F 12 (*Escherichia coli*). Filamentous phage with single-stranded DNA (*see* fd).

G (*Bacillus megaterium*). Large icosahedral phage with contractile tail. The sheath, 455 nm, contracts to 188 nm. 41% (G+C). (Donelli *et al.*, 1972.)

GA (*Escherichia coli*). Member of group II of RNA phages. The coat protein has N-terminal Ala- and C-terminal -(Tyr,Phe)Ala. (Miyake *et al.*, 1971.)

GA/1 (*Bacillus stearothermophilus* and *B. subtilis*). Phage with oblong head and short noncontractile tail with collar and three pins.

GA/2 (*Bacillus subtilis*). Defective phage, possibly identical to PBSX.

gh-1 (*Pseudomonas putida*). Virus contains 31 S DNA of 23×10^6 mol. wt., containing 57% (G+C).

GH 5 (*Bacillus stearothermophilus*). Thermophilic phage; buoyant density in CsCl 1.473 g/ml. (Humbert and Fields, 1972.)

GH 8 (*Bacillus stearothermophilus*). Thermophilic phage of buoyant density in CsCl 1.506 g/ml. The hexagonal particle has a diameter of 100 nm and a 330 nm tail. (Humbert and Fields, 1972.)

GR (*Escherichia coli*). Member of group I of RNA phages (*see* f 2).

GT 1–5 (*Bacillus thuringiensis*). Five temperate phages.

GT 234 (*Streptococcus*). Temperate transducing phage. Morphologically like A 25 and serologically related to it. (Colón *et al.*, 1971.)

GV 1–6 (*Bacillus thuringiensis*). Six virulent phages of three morphological types.

γ (*Bacillus arthracis*). Contains 36% (G + C).

γ (2) (*Escherichia coli*). Similar size to λ, with flexuous tail with a few fine fibers. (Gratia, 1973.)

H (*Pasteurella pestis*). Almost identical to I, II (*Escherichia coli*). (Brunovskis *et al.*, 1973.)

HM 2, 3 (*Clostridium saccharoperbutylacetonicum*). Contain, respectively, 35 and 30% (G+C).

HP 1 (*Haemophilus influenzae*) (mutants HP 1 cl and c2). Temperate phage of high transfection efficiency (10^{-3}), related to S 2. Particles of 52 × 50 nm with a 19 × 122 nm contractile tail. Contains DNA of 20 × 10^6 daltons with cohesive ends. (Notani *et al.*, 1973; Boling *et al.*, 1973.)

HR (*Escherichia coli*). Filamentous 6 × 800 nm particle; density 1.31.

If 1, 2 (*Salmonella typhimurium* and *Escherichia coli*). Filamentous particles of 5.5 × 1300 nm, longer than the Ff group (e.g., fd). These phages adsorb specifically to I-pili and are thus not sex-specific, in contrast to members of the Ff group and most RNA phages. Buoyant density in CsCl is 1.30 g/ml; 45 S; particle weight 25 × 10^6. The DNA is 1.5 times longer than that of fd (about 3 × 10^6 daltons). Part of the DNA is self-complementary. A/G/T/C = 27/23/28/22. The coat protein consists of 49 amino acids, with seven exchanges compared to fd. There are also a few molecules of an A protein. (Meynell and Lawn, 1968; Wiseman *et al.*, 1972; Kay and Wakefield, 1972.)

IKe (*Escherichia coli* and *Salmonella typhimurium*). Filamentous particles of 6.6 × 900–1300 nm. The buoyant density of the phage in CsCl is 1.286 ml, that of the single-stranded DNA 1.7218. The phage is sex-factor specific and can be differentiated from If in terms of this specificity, as well as serologically. (Khatoon *et al.*, 1972.)

I 3 (*Mycobacterium smegmatis*). Transducing phage. Isometric 80 nm diameter particle with visible capsomeres, and an 80 nm tail which contracts to 48 nm. (Kozloff *et al.*, 1972.)

K-phages (*Escherichia coli*, capsular strains). Eleven strains, resemble P 22 with diameter varying from 45 to 65 nm; one has a long contractile tail (56 × 88 nm diameter head, 100 nm tail), and one a long noncontractile tail (50 × 56 nm head, 168 nm tail). All have spikes and no fibers. (Stirm and Freund-Mölbert, 1971.)

KJ (*Escherichia coli*). Member of group II of RNA phages. (Miyake *et al.*, 1971.)

κ (*Serratia narcescens*). Temperate phage containing 54% (G+C).

K 1 (*Streptomyces coelicolor*). Particles with long noncontractile tail. (Coyette and Calberg-Bacq, 1967.)

L (*Salmonella typhimurium*). Transducing phage related to P 22. Buoyant density in CsCl is 1.51 g/ml.

Lambda, *see* λ.

LH II (L II) BNV 6–1, 6–2 (*Agrobacterium tumefaciens*). Hexagonal
head (72 nm diameter) and long (235 nm) flexuous tail with six appendages near end (591 S); particle weight 71×10^6; buoyant
density in CsCl 1.511 g/ml. (Manasse *et al.,* 1972.)

LH II (L II) BV 7–1, 7–2, very similar to the above two phages.

LPP 1 and LPP 2 (*Lyngbya, Plectonema,* and *Phormidium,* filamentous genera of blue-green algae, all not susceptible to AS 1).
LPP 1 and LPP 2 are morphologically similar but serologically unrelated. Particles of 58 nm diameter, with short, forked tails (10–20
$\times$15 nm), containing DNA of 29×10^6 mol. wt. (34 S), 13.2 μm
long, and containing 54% (G+C). (Sherman and Haselkorn, 1970.)

LT 2 (*Salmonella typhimurium*). Similar to L.

LV 1 (*Agrobacterium tumefaciens*) (very similar to or identical with ω,
PB 2A, PS 8). Particles with hexagonal head of 70 nm diameter
with flexuous tail of 200 nm. They contain 34.5 S DNA (no nicks),
34×10^6 mol. wt., 14.2 μm long; buoyant density in CsCl 1.505;
57% (G+C). The main proteins have molecular weights of 48×10^3
(50%), 30×10^3 (30%), 16×10^3 (16%), and 69×10^3 (4%). The
etiological role of phages of this type in crowngall tumors of plants
is very dubious, in contrast to that of their hosts, *Agrobacterium
tumefacieus*. (de Ley *et al.,* 1972.)

λ (*Escherichia coli*). Classical prototype of lysogenic (temperate)
phages. Icosahedral particles of 54 nm diameter with evident
capsomeres, carrying a thin noncontractile tail (15 $\times$ 150 nm) with
fine cross-striation and a thin fiber (2 $\times$ 25 nm) at the end. The
particle weight is 60×10^6 (416 S).The tail weight is 6.5×10^6. The
particle weights of head (without the DNA) and tail are 18 and 6 $\times$
10^6 (114 S and 43 S). The phage contains one molecule of double-
stranded DNA (34 S) of 30×10^6 daltons and 17.2 μm contour
length. The composition is 49% (G+C). The DNA has cohesive
ends (12 nucleotide pairs long, between the arrows) and the sequence of 25 base pairs in the terminal areas are known:

```
              ↓
5' –GTTACGGGGCGGCGACCTCGCGGGT–  light strand
3'         –CCCGCCGCTGGAGCGCCCA–  denser strand
                        ↑
```

The DNA of λ yields upon shearing two halves of unequal (G+C)
content, the so-called left-hand portion being denser and higher in
(G+C) than the right (55 *vs.* 45%). There is also a difference in the

density of the two strands, but this difference is less than in many other phages.

The main proteins have been identified as composing the head (38×10^3 daltons, 60% or 540 molecules), the tail (31×10^3 daltons, 19%), the tail fiber (130×10^3 daltons), and a protein playing an internal role, particularly during maturation (12×10^3, 19%, 550 molecules per particle). Mutant capsids, termed "petit," lack that protein. There are also six minor protein components of $79\text{-}14 \times 10^3$ daltons. At least 18 genes are involved in the morphogenesis of λ, 7 with head formation and the rest with tail assembly. The endolysin, the product of gene R, has been purified and sequenced (157 residues, one cysteine). It is unrelated to the T-even phage lysozymes.

Many more or less closely related strains of λ are known. These are, in order of diminishingly close relationship, 82 and 434, 21, 424, and 80. They are listed separately in this catalogue. (Phage 186 is related to P 2, 299, D, and N 1, not to λ.) These and others are defective mutants, carrying varying amounts of the host's gal and bio gene. Many of them differ in molecular weight, contour length, and composition. (For amino acid composition of pure protein components of λ, see Table 5.) (Buchwald *et al.*, 1970; Weigel *et al.*, 1973; Murialdo and Siminovitch, 1972.)

M (*Proteus morgani*). 49% (G+C).

MG 40 (*Salmonella typhimurium*). Similar to L.

Mp (*Aerobacter aerogenes, Escherichia coli,* and *Klebsiella pneumoniae, not Salmonella, Proteus, Serratia* spp.). Hexagonal 62 nm head, flexuous tail of 6×165 nm. Contains DNA of 23×10^6 mol. wt., 50% (G+C). (Souza *et al.*, 1972.)

MP 1, 2 (*Methanomonas methylovora*). Similar to MP 3.

MP 3 (*Methanomonas methylovora*). Particles of about 100 nm diameter with tails of 30×100 nm and base plates. Contains DNA of 35% (G+C). (Oki *et al.*, 1972.)

MS 2 (*Escherichia coli*). Member of group I of RNA phages (*see* f 2).

MSP 8 (*Streptomyces griseus*). 70% (G+C).

MU 1 (or μ 1 or only MU) (*Escherichia coli*). A temperate phage of appearance and size similar to λ but in density and DNA content more similar to defective λ strains; serologically not related to λ. The DNA is 12.9 μm long, of 30.7 S, 25×10^6 mol. wt., and 51%

(G+C), almost the same as the DNA of the host. The phage has a unique propensity for stable integration at many positions, and for increased mutation frequency. (Martuscelli *et al.,* 1971.)

Mushroom viruses, *see* Section B (plant viruses).

MY (*Escherichia coli*). Member of group I of RNA phages (*See* f 2).

MVG 51 (*Acholeplasma laidlawii*). Rod-shaped virus, not enveloped, similar to but different from MVL 1, MVL 52. (Liss and Maniloff, 1971.)

MV L 1 (*Acholeplasma laidlawii*) (Mycoplasmatales virus-laidlawii). Bacilliform particles (average 14 × 90 nm). Hexagons forming a helix. The virus is ether resistant and relatively heat stable. It contains DNA. (Bruce *et al.,* 1972; Milne *et al.,* 1972.)

MV L 2 (*Acholeplasma laidlawii*). Spherical particles averaging 80 nm diameter which are enveloped and ether sensitive. Probably contains DNA. (Gourlay *et al.,* 1971; Gourlay *et al.,* 1973.)

MV L 3 (*Acholeplasma laidlawii*). Polyhedral, possibly hexagonal particles of 54 nm diameter. This virus is serologically and in host range specificity different from MV L 1 and 2.

MV L 52 (*Acholeplasma laidlawii*), *see* MVG 51. (Liss and Maniloff, 1971.)

MX 1 (*Micrococcus xanthus*). Typical phage with contractile tail. (Burchard and Voelz, 1972.)

M 12 (*Escherichia coli*). Member of group I of RNA phages (*see* f 2).

M 13 (*Escherichia coli*). Filamentous particles with single-stranded DNA, closely related to fd. Length 850–900 nm, buoyant density in CsCl 1.29 g/ml. The DNA has a molecular weight of 2×10^6. A/G/T/C = 23/21/36/20. The coat protein has the same amino acid composition and presumably sequence as fd. (Henry and Brinton, 1971.)

M 51 (*Brucella* spp.). Morphologically but not serologically identical to Tbilisi phage.

μ (*Serratia narcescens*). Probably identical with η.

μ 1 (*Escherichia coli*), *see* MU 1.

μ 2 (*Escherichia coli*). Member of group II of RNA phages (Miyake *et al.,* 1971.)

μ **4** (*Bacillus stearothermophilus*). Polyhedral particle of 55 nm diameter with long tail (7 × 225 nm) lacking base plate and fibers. $A_{260/280}$ = 1.57. Contains DNA of 33 S, 26 × 10^6 mol. wt., density 1.719 g/ml; 58 or 46% (G+C). The strands can be separated on CsCl gradients. (Rabussay *et al.*, 1970.)

μ **4** (*Bacillus subtilis*). Unusually small (10 nm diameter) tailless particle.

NC MB 384, 385 (*Flavobacterium, Cytophaga* spp.). Particles with long noncontractile tail. 31% (G+C). (Bradley, 1967.)

NH (*Escherichia coli*). Member of group III of RNA phages (*see* Qβ).

NM (*Escherichia coli*). Member of group III of RNA phages (*see* Qβ).

NT 1–4 (*Rhizobium trifolii*). NT 1, particles of 62 nm diameter with 12 × 140 nm tail; NT 2, 60 nm diameter with 12 × 170 nm tail; NT 3, 57 nm diameter with 15 × 130 nm tail; NT 4, 60 nm diameter with 9 × 110 nm tail; all noncontractile tails. (Barnet, 1972.)

N 1 (Blue-green algae; filamentous, N-fixing species, e.g., *Nostoc muscorum*) (resembles T-even phages). Particles with 61 nm diameter head, 100 nm long contractile tail (539 S). Flexuous fibers are attached to the neck of the virion. The phage contains DNA of 1.69 g/ml buoyant density in CsCl; 39 S; 37% (G+C); 43 × 10^6 mol. wt; 17.2 μm long. At least 19 proteins of molecular weights 87–13 × 10^3 have been detected. (Adolph and Haselkorn, 1971, 1973.)

N 1 (*Micrococcus lysodeicticus* and *Escherichia coli*). Temperate phage. Similar and related to 186. DNA of 30 × 10^6 dalton molecular weight, with cohesive ends, 65% (G+C).

N 3 (*Haemophilus influenzae*). Particles with 60 nm diameter head and 200 nm noncontractile tail lacking base plate and fiber. (Unrelated to HP 1, etc.)

N 4 (*Escherichia coli*) (similar to T 3, T 7). Icosahedral particles of 70 nm diameter; 436 S; 83 × 10^6 particle weight; with base plate and noncontractile tail. The DNA (48%) is 23 μm long, 45 × 10^6 mol. wt., 41 S, and contains 44% (G+C). Ten proteins, of molecular weights 31,000 to 92,000, were detected. (Sinha *et al.*, 1973.)

N 5, N 6 (*Micrococcus lysodeicticus*). Particles similar to λ (*E. coli*), containing 30 × 10^6 dalton DNA with cohesive ends. (N 6: 70% (G+C).)

ω (*Agrobacterium tumefaciens*) (closely related if not identical to LV 1, R 4, PS 8, PB 2A), *see* LV 1.

PB 1 (*Pseudomonas aeruginosa*). Octahedral particle of 75 nm diameter with 150 nm contractile tail, no base plate, and four 60 nm tail fibers folded back against the sheath. The DNA, 25 μm long, occupies 45% of head space. (Bradley, 1966.)

PB 2 (*Pseudomonas syringae*). Particles with elongated head (70 × 100 nm), and noncontractile tail of 175 nm. (Similar to PP 4.)

PB 2 (*Escherichia coli*). The phage is 610 S, 68 × 10⁶ particle weight, buoyant density in CsCl 1.44 g/ml. It contains DNA of T_m 87°C. (Velikodvorskaya *et al.*, 1972.)

PB 2A (*Agrobacterium tumefaciens*). Identical with ω, PS 8, and LV 1. Buoyant density in CsCl is 1.505 g/ml, 56% (G+C) (*see* LV 1).

PB 6, 7, 8, 9, 10, 29, 84, 1197 (*Pseudomonas aeruginosa*). Contain DNA of 31 S, 23 × 10⁶ mol. wt. (Bradley, 1966; Bartell and Orr, 1969; Bartell *et al.*, 1971.)

PBP 1 (*Bacillus pumilus*). Transducing phage infecting only flagellated strains of bacteria. Head of 65 nm diameter and 200 nm noncontractile tail with flexuous fibers. (Lovett, 1972.)

PBSX (*Bacillus subtilis*) (also called PBSH and GA/2). A defective phage carrying only host DNA. The hexagonal particles have a diameter of 41 nm; a contractile tail of 18 × 196 nm with 70 nm tail fibers; 160 S; 1.375 g/ml buoyant density in CsCl. The DNA (of the host) is linear and of 9–12 × 10⁶ mol. wt., 23 S, and 43% (G+C); its length is 4.7 μm. (Okamoto *et al.*, 1968; Haas and Yoshikawa, 1969.)

PBS 1 (*Bacillus subtilis*). Particle weight 200 × 10⁶ (72 S); 28% (G+C), containing U instead of T. Infects only flagellated strains.

PBS 2 (*Bacillus subtilis*). DNA of 28% (G+C); contains U instead of T (also glucose). (Price and Cook, 1972.)

PBV 1 and PBV 3 (*Penicillium brevicompactum;* infectious for *E. coli*). Icosahedral 45 nm diameter particle with long noncontractile tail. Buoyant density in CsCl is 1.48 g/ml for PBV 1 and 1.51 for PBV 3. Contains linear DNA. (Tikhonenko *et al.*, 1973).

PBV 2 (*Penicillium brevicompactum;* infectious for *E. coli*). Icosahedral particles of 53 nm diameter with a short tail. Buoyant density in CsCl is 1.48 g/ml; 610 S, 68 × 10⁶ particle weight; contains 43% of linear DNA of 25.2 × 10⁶ mol. wt. (30 S), 44% (G+C).

Pc (*Pseudomonas aeruginosa*). Particle with 60 nm head, 165 nm non-contractile tail with knob at end. (Bradley, 1966.)

PcV (*Penicillium chrysogenum*). Icosahedral particles of 37 nm diameter, 150 S, buoyant density in CsCl 1.35 g/ml; particle weight 13×10^6. Contains about 13% double-stranded RNA of 1.89, 1.99, and 2.8×10^6 mol. wt. (Wood and Bozarth, 1972.)

Pf 1 (*Pseudomonas aeruginosa,* K strain). Filamentous phage, 1900 nm long; adsorbs to pili, but not male-specific. Contains 12% single-stranded DNA (Takeya and Amako, 1966.)

Pf 2 (*Pseudomonas aeruginosa*). Filamentous phage indistinguishable from Pf 1 in several respects. (Minamishima *et al.,* 1968.)

PK (*Escherichia coli* and *Bacillus subtilis*). Mutant of P2. (Jesaitis and Hutton, 1963.)

pKc (*Bacillus subtilis*). 63 S DNA containing 35% (G+C).

PL 25 (*Proteus morganii,* Providence strains). Particles of 485 S, 57×10^6 particle weight, containing 26×10^6 mol. wt. DNA, 12.6 μm long (similar to P 22 of *Salmonella*). (Coetzee *et al.,* 1966.)

PL 26 (*Proteus morganii,* Providence strains). 42% (G+C). (Coetzee *et al.,* 1966.)

PL 27 (*Proteus morganii,* Providence strains). 58×10^6 DNA. (Coetzee *et al.,* 1966.)

PLT 22 (*Salmonella typhimurium*). Temperate phage.

PM 2 (*Pseudomonas* BAL-31). Lipid-containing icosahedral particle of 62 nm diameter, particle weight 58×10^6 daltons, containing circular superhelical 6×10^6 dalton DNA of 42% (G+C). The phage contains 13% lipid (not enough for continuous lipid bilayer), mostly (12%) phospholipid; 75% protein; 11% DNA; and traces of carbohydrate. The proteins have molecular weights of 43,000 (190 molecules), 32,000 (160 molecules), 12,000 (730 molecules, lipoprotein), and 5000 (660 molecules, glycolipoprotein). (Harrison *et al.,* 1971.)

PO 2, PO 4 (*Pseudomonas aeruginosa*). Phages adsorb to pili. Hexagonal particle of 58 nm diameter with 186 nm noncontractile tail and bar-shaped basal structure. Same appearance as PP 4, PS 4, which probably are not pilus-phages. (Bradley, 1973.)

PP 1 (*Pseudomonas aeruginosa*). Probably identical with PB 1.

PP 4 (*Pseudomonas aeruginosa*). Probably octahedral particles of 60 nm diameter, 195 nm noncontractile tail with cross at end (like PS 4). (Bradley, 1966.)

PP 7 (*Pseudomonas aeruginosa*). Isometric particles of 25 nm diameter which adsorb to polar pili and contain RNA (similar to *E. coli* RNA phages). (Bradley, 1972, 1973.)

PR 590a (*Agrobacterium radiobacter*). Particles with short non-contractile tail. (Roslycky *et al.*, 1963.)

PR 1001 (*Agrobacterium radiobacter*). 53% (G+C). (Roslycky *et al.*, 1963.)

PRM 1 (*Rhizobium meliloti*). 49% (G+C).

PS 1 (*Penicillium stoloniferum*). Mycophages containing double-stranded RNA (interferon stimulator). Particles of 30 nm diameter. (van Frank *et al.*, 1971.)

PS 4 (*Pseudomonas syringae*). Phage resembles PP 4.

PS 8 (*Agrobacterium tumefaciens*). Temperate phage, identical to PB 2A and LV 1 (*see* LV 1).

PS 192 (*Agrobacterium radiobacter*). Phage resembles PR 1001. (Roslycky *et al.*, 1963.)

PsR 1012 (*Agrobacterium radiobacter*). Phage resembles PR 1001. (Roslycky *et al.*, 1963.)

PSVf (*Penicillium stoloniferum*) (serologically distinct from PSVs). Isometric particles of 34 nm diameter containing double-stranded RNA of 0.99, 0.89, and 0.23 $\times$ 10^6 mol. wt., separately encapsidated. (Buck and Kempson-Jones, 1973.)

PSVs (*Penicillium stoloniferum*) (serologically distinct from PSVf). Isometric particles of 34 nm diameter of 66, 87, 101, and 113 S, containing, respectively, no RNA, single-stranded RNA (9%), double-stranded RNA (16%), and both types of RNA (24%). The molecular weights of the single-stranded RNAs of the two components of each of these fractions are 0.47 and 0.56 $\times$ 10^6. (Buck and Kempson-Jones, 1973.)

P 0362 (*Agrobacterium tumefaciens*). Defective particles of 65 nm diameter and straight 130 nm tail. DNA of 25 $\times$ 10^6 mol. wt., buoyant density in CsCl 1.458 g/ml, 56% (G+C); also lower T_m and different protein pattern than the LV 1 group. (de Ley *et al.*, 1972.)

P 1 (*Salmonella, Escherichia coli,* etc.). Generalized transducing phage. Icosahedral particle of 65 nm diameter with noncontractile tail of 20 × 200 nm. Particle weight 90 × 10⁶. Molecular weight of the DNA 60 × 10⁶, contour length 32 μm. The virus does not integrate its DNA into the host chromosome, but resides in the cell as a plasmid. Specific restriction and modification systems were first studied in this phage. The DNA contains 0.3% 6-methyladenine and half as much 5-methylcytosine. (Rosner, 1972; Ikeda and Tomizawa, 1965.)

P 1c3, mutant of P 1. (Scott and Shuster, 1973.)

P1kc (*Escherichia coli*). Particle of 90 nm diameter with 20 × 220 nm contractile tail; buoyant density 1.47 g/ml in CsCl. The DNA contains 46% (G+C).

P 2 (*Salmonella* and *Escherichia coli*). Temperate phage. Polyhedral, probably icosahedral particles of 58 nm diameter with a cylindrical contractile tail of 17 × 135 nm, with thin tail fibers, 40–50 nm long. The particle weight is 58 × 10⁶.

The DNA (38%) has a molecular weight of 22 × 10⁶. Its length is 13.2 μm. It is linear and nonpermuted, with cohesive ends consisting of 19 single-stranded nucleotides. It coheres with 186 and 299, even though its cohesive sequences differ slightly (by one nucleotide). The cohesive sequences of P 2 and P 4 are identical, but quite different from those of unrelated λ.

The head consists to 90% of the major capsid protein and contains at least six minor components. The major protein is cleaved from 44,000 to 36,000 daltons in the course of phage maturation, coincident with release of two of the minor proteins derived from the same gene (N). There are also at least four tail proteins. (Lengyel *et al.,* 1973; Barrett *et al.,* 1973; Bertani and Bertani, 1971; Murray and Murray, 1973.)

P 3 (*Salmonella potsdam*). Hexagonal head of 48 × 55 nm with 12 × 118 nm tail, the sheath of which contracts to 42 nm, exposing the 5.5 nm core. Six short fibers at the end of the core are evident. The phage is very heat resistant. (Nutter *et al.,* 1970.)

P 4 (*Salmonella potsdam*). Hexagonal head of 48 × 55 nm with short tail (9 × 15 nm). (Nutter *et al.,* 1970.)

P 4 (*Escherichia coli*). A defective satellite of P 2. The isometric particles have a diameter of 40 nm and a contractile tail very similar if not identical to that of P 2 (17 × 135 nm), with thin 45-nm-long fibers. The DNA has the same cohesive ends as that of P 2, but is only one-third as long, 3.9 μm, molecular weight about 7×10^6 (the capacity of the head is also one-third of that of P 2). There is no detectable homology (< 1%) between the DNA of P 2 and P 4. The proteins of P 4 appear to be the same as those of P 2. (Barrett *et al.*, 1973.)

P 9a (*Salmonella potsdam*). Very similar to P 3. (Nutter *et al.*, 1970.)

P 9c (*Salmonella potsdam*). Very similar to P 4. (Nutter *et al.*, 1970.)

P 10 (*Salmonella potsdam*) (serologically related to P 3, P 9a). Hexagonal head of 48×55 nm with 12×95 nm helical tail, which contracts to 38 nm, exposing 6 nm core. Base plate carrying six long straight fibers. Very heat sensitive. (Nutter *et al.*, 1970.)

P 11 (*Staphylococcus aureus*). General transducing phage. (Novick, 1967.)

P 11-M 15 (*Staphylococcus aureus*). A virulent mutant of the temperate phage P 11. Particles of 50–60 nm diameter, 445 S, and 67×10^6 dalton particle weight, with 150 nm flexuous non-contractile tail. The phage contains 49% DNA of 33×10^6 mol. wt., lacking cohesive ends or nicks. (Brown *et al.*, 1972.)

P 22 (*Salmonella*). Temperate general transducing phage (which can integrate at several sites—not as many as MU 1). Isometric 60 nm diameter particles with short six-pin tail assembly. The DNA is 26×10^6 daltons, 13 μm long, and of a buoyant density in CsCl of 1.7069 g/ml. It is, like those of P 1 and the T-even phages, circularly permuted and terminally redundant. The DNA contains small amounts of 6-methyladenine, which vary in different hosts. It contains 49% (G+C).

The main head protein (55×10^3 daltons) forms proheads in conjunction with a scaffolding protein (42×10^3 daltons) which leaves the maturing phage. Minor proteins of the head are 94, 67, 50, and 18×10^3 daltons. Those of the short tail assembly and pins are 23 and 76×10^3 daltons. The full heads, proheads, and empty heads have 500 S, 240 S, and 170 S. (King *et al.*, 1973.)

P 42 D (*Staphylococcus* B). Particles of 55 nm diameter with 230 nm tails.

P 52 A (*Staphylococcus* B). Particles of 50 nm diameter with 150 nm tails.

P 8149 (*Agrobacterium radiobacter*). Defective phage not related to

LV 1 group of crowngall-associated factors. Buoyant density in CsCl is 1.510 g/ml. Bipyramidal particles with 40 nm diameter head and short tail, DNA of 10×10^6 mol. wt., 60% (G+C). (de Ley *et al.*, 1972.)

Qβ (*Escherichia coli*). Prototype of group III RNA phages. This virus is very similar in most of its properties to the phages of group I, although serologically these groups are unrelated. The isometric particles are of about 25 nm diameter; 80 S; 4×10^6 dalton particle weight. They contain one molecule of RNA of probably 1.2×10^6 molecular weight, which, like all phage RNAs, is able to infect spheroblasts.

As for the other RNA phages, the 5'- and 3'-ends are pppGpGpG- and -CpCpCpA. The 3'-terminal A of this, as of other phage RNAs, is not necessary for infectivity, and it is regenerated in the progeny of deadenylated phage. The nucleotide sequence of this RNA is known to about 20% (Figure 5). There is some similarity in nucleotide sequences between this RNA and those of group I phages (Figure 3).

The coat protein of Qβ consists of 131 amino acids and its sequence shows some similarities to those of group I phages (Figure 4). It lacks histidine, methionine, and tryptophan. Besides the 180 molecules of coat protein building up the phage particle, there is one molecule (or very few) of the A protein or maturation protein which is essential for the integrity of the phage, as well as during the infection process. This protein has a molecular weight of 44,000, and the N-terminal sequence (F-Met)-Pro-Lys-Leu-Pro-.

There is also generally found a small amount of an additional protein which results from read-through of a termination codon, and represents the coat protein plus additional $\sim 23,000$ mol. wt. protein material.

Besides coding for the coat and maturation proteins, Qβ RNA also codes for a peptide chain of about 65,000 which in the host combines with three host protein factors of molecular weights of 72,000, 45,000, and 35,000 daltons to make up the Qβ-specific RNA polymerase (or replicase). Its N-terminal sequence is (F-Met)-Ser-Lys-Thr-Ala-. (Miyake *et al.*, 1971; Weissmann *et al.*, 1973; Königsberg *et al.*, 1970.)

R (*Salmonella typhimurium*). Particles resemble X 174 (12 "tails").

R 1, R 2 (*Streptomyces coelicolor*). Typical particles with long non-contractile tail. (Coyette and Calberg-Bacq, 1967.)

R 4 (*Agrobacterium tumefaciens,* which transforms plant cells, and thus produces crowngall) (related to PS 8, PB 2A, LV 1, and ω). Polyhedral head of 65 nm diameter with flexuous tail of 10×210 nm. Buoyant density in CsCl 1.51 g/ml. DNA of 34 S, 30×10^6 mol. wt., buoyant density in CsCl 1.718 g/ml, 59% (G+C). The phage contains four major proteins of 72, 45, 28, and 14.5×10^3 mol. wt. The phage probably plays no major role in crowngall formation. (Adler and Pootjes, 1972.)

RI (*Nocardia restrictus*). Hexagonal 75-nm-long particle with long flexuous noncontractile tail and 10×330 nm tail. (DNA not characterized.)

R 17 (*Escherichia coli*). Much studied member of group I of RNA phages (*see* f 2).

R 23 (*Escherichia coli*). Member of group I of RNA phages (*see* f 2). This phage completely dominates RNA synthesis in the host. (Watanabe *et al., 1968.*)

SA (*Staphylococcus pyogenes*). Contains DNA of 34% (G+C).

SBX-1 (*Xanthomonas* sp. 1, growing in soybeans). The polyhedral head is elongated (80×83 nm diameter) and carries a tail of 112 nm, with base plate and spikes. The DNA has a buoyant density in CsCl of 1.709 g/ml, 49.5% (G+C), compared to the host's 55.4% (G+C). (Dunleavy and Urs, 1973.)

S$_D$ (*Escherichia coli* SK). Icosahedral head of 59 nm diameter and short (20×20 nm) tail. Particle weight is 118×10^6, 780 S, buoyant density in CsCl 1.45 g/ml. The DNA (43%) of 51 S, 58×10^6 mol. wt., is 43% (G+C) (1.700 g/ml buoyant density in CsCl). (Kisseleva and Tikhonenko, 1972.)

SD (*Escherichia coli*). Member of group II of RNA phages. The coat protein has N-terminal Ala- and C-terminal -(Tyr, Phe)Ala. (Miyake *et al., 1971.*)

Si 1 (*Spirillum itersonii*). Large icosahedral phage with 26×10^6 dalton DNA containing 53% (G+C).

SM 1 (*Synechococcus* and other unicellular forms of blue-green algae only). Icosahedral particle of 67 nm diameter, 100×10^6 dalton particle weight (820 S); a very short collar and thin appendage (tail). The 48 S DNA is of 59×10^6 dalton molecular weight, and 67% (G+C). The virus contains twelve proteins, two of which (of

40,000 and 25,000) contain 80% of the sulfur. (Mackenzie and Haselkorn, 1972.)

SM 2, *see* under SMP.

SM 4 (*Serratia* spp.). Similar to P 22, with complex tail assembly.

SMP, SM 2 (*Serratia narcescens,* as well as *Salmonella, Escherichia,* etc.). SMP, SM 2 are among the largest known phages, with a head of 135 nm diameter (almost twice the volume of T 2) and a contractile tail of 28 × 235 nm. The tail in extended form resembles the stacked disk form of TMV protein.

SP (*Escherichia coli*). Member of group IV of RNA phages. (Miyake *et al.,* 1971.)

SPX (*Bacillus subtilis*). Defective phage containing 43% (G+C).

SPα (*Bacillus subtilis*). Defective phage containing 43% (G+C).

SPO 1 (*Bacillus subtilis*). Virulent phage related to SP 82. Contains 100 × 10⁶ mol. wt. DNA, 54 S, of 44% (G+C), and with hydroxymethyl-U instead of T. (Levner and Cozzarelli, 1972.)

SPO 2 (*Bacillus subtilis*). Temperate phage. Similar but genetically unrelated to 105, although there is some serological cross-reactivity. Icosahedral particles of 50 nm diameter with 177 nm tail with complex six-pronged tail tip structure. Contains 25 × 10⁶ mol. wt. DNA, with cohesive ends, 13 μm long, carrying 18 complementation groups. (Rutberg *et al.,* 1972.)

SPP 1 (*Bacillus subtilis*). Closely related to SPO 2. Hexagonal head of 50 nm diameter with 177-nm-long tail. The DNA of 25 × 10⁶ mol. wt. has no single-strand breaks; however, it has cohesive ends. The strands of this DNA can be separated on the basis of different densities (1.713 and 1.725 g/ml) in CsCl, and contain, respectively, 43 and 57% pyrimidines. the buoyant density of the duplex DNA is 1.7003. This is the most infective DNA known, 5–6 × 10³ molecules being able to initiate a plaque. (Riva, 1969.)

SP 3 (*Bacillus subtilis*). Large phage of 110 nm diameter with 22 × 260 nm tail sheath, that contracts to 150 nm. Its DNA is of 69 S, 150 × 10⁶ mol. wt., and 35% (G+C). (Eiserling and Romig, 1962.)

SP 5 (*Bacillus licheniformis*). Contains an unusual base, probably 5-hydroxymethyl-U.

SP 8 (*Bacillus subtilis*). Contains DNA of 69 × 10⁶ mol. wt. (54 S), the strands of which can be separated because of different density (57 and 43% pyrimidines, with densities in CsCl of 1.725 and 1.713 g/ml, respectively). The DNA is 39% (G+C) and contains 5-hydroxymethyl-U (and glucose?). (Truffaut *et al.*, 1970.)

SP 10 (*Bacillus subtilis*). DNA contains 44% (G+C).

SP 15 (*Bacillus subtilis*). Large general transducing phage of many peculiarities. A/G/T/C = 29/21/17/21, with 12% 5-(4′,5′-dihydroxypentyl)-U. The DNA also contains alkali-sensitive ester bonds and glucose. Its density is unusually high (1.761 g/ml) and its T_m low (61.5%). It infects only flagellated strains of bacteria. (Marmur *et al.*, 1972.)

SP 50 (*Bacillus subtilis*). Contains 100×10^6 mol. wt. DNA (54 S), 50 μm long, with random interruption of both strands; it is 42% (G+C). (Truffaut *et al.*, 1970.)

SP 60 (*Bacillus subtilis*). Contains 130×10^6 mol. wt. DNA (63 S) of 43% (G+C), with 5-hydroxymethyl-U instead of T.

SP 70, 80, 90, 100 (*Bacillus subtilis*) (related to PBS 1, 2).

SP 82 (G) (*Bacillus subtilis*) (related to SPO 1). Similar to T 4 in size and structure. Contains 130×10^6 mol. wt. DNA, 39% (G+C), with 5-hydroxymethyl-U instead of T. (Truffaut *et al.*, 1970.)

SP 105 (*Bacillus subtilis*). DNA of 49 S, 63×10^6 mol. wt.

ST (*Escherichia coli*). Member of group III of RNA phages (*see* Qβ).

ST (*Rhizobium trifolii*). (Barnet, 1972.)

SW (*Escherichia coli*). Member of group II of RNA phages. (Miyake *et al.*, 1971.)

SW (*Bacillus subtilis*). Icosahedral head of 101 nm diameter with long contractile tail (22×172 nm), 910 S; 292×10^6 in particle weight; buoyant density in CsCl 1.52 g/ml. The linear DNA is of 62 S, 127×10^6 mol. wt., and 45% (G+C). The T is replaced by 5-hydroxymethyl-U (Petrovsky *et al.*, 1970.)

S 1 (*Synechococcus* strain NRC-1, a unicellular blue-green alga). Head of 50 nm diameter and 140 nm noncontractile tail; 353 S; buoyant density in CsCl 1.501 g/ml. The DNA is of 31 S and 13.3 μm length, 25×10^6 mol. wt., with 72% (G+C). Thirteen proteins were detected, the main capsid proteins having molecular weights of

39,000 (63%), 11,000 (7%), and 10,000 (11%). Almost all properties are very similar to those of λ. (Adolph and Haselkorn, 1973.)

S 2 (*Hemophilus influenzae*) (related to HP 1). Particles of 49 × 46 nm with 19 × 117 nm contractile tail. Contains 20 × 10⁶ mol. wt. DNA with cohesive ends. (Boling *et al.*, 1973.)

S 13 (*Escherichia coli*). Member of X 174 group of single-stranded DNA phages. Serologically related to X 174 with much homology in DNA sequences, but little complete homology. Only one of the eight proteins is identical in the two phages. (Poljak and Suruda, 1969; Godson, 1973.)

S 24 V (*Serratia*). 58% (G+C).

S 708 (*Brucella* spp.). Morphologically but not serologically identical to Tbilisi phage. (Morris *et al.*, 1973.)

Tbilisi (*Brucella abortus*) Hexagonal icosahedral head (∼65 nm diameter) and short tail. Contains DNA of 49% (G+C). (*See also* A 422, M 51, and S 708.)

t (*Serratia narcescens*). Temperate phage with DNA of 56% (G+C).

TP1C, TP 8, TP 12 (*Bacillus stearothermophilus*). Temperate phages.

TP 84 (*Bacillus stearothermophilus*). Typical particle (436 S) of 50 × 10⁶ daltons, with 37 × 64 nm head and 10 × 150 nm tail. The DNA of 30 S and 32 × 10⁶ mol. wt. contains 42% (G+C). (Kizer and Saunders, 1972.)

TSP 1 (*Bacillus subtilis*). Temperature-sensitive strain, growing only above 50°C. Hexagonal head 90 nm in diameter and 200-nm-long contractile tail, rigid when contracted. The 56 × 10⁶ mol. wt. DNA contains 45% (G+C). (LaMontagne and McDonald, 1972.)

Tφ 3 (*Bacillus stearothermophilus*). The DNA of 38 S is 11.7 μm long, 22.5 × 10⁶ mol. wt., and 40% (G+C). (Egbert, 1972.)

T 1 (*Escherichia coli*). Icosahedral head of 50 nm diameter, with a long noncontractile tail (10 × 150 nm). Its linear double-stranded DNA (34 S) has a molecular weight of about 30 × 10⁶. It is terminally redundant, without circular permutation, and lacking cohesive ends. The DNA has a contour length of 16 μm. Its composition is 47% (G+C). (Male and Christensen, 1970.)

T 2 (*Escherichia coli*). In almost all respects, T 2 is very similar to or identical with T 4 and T 6, and the general features of these three phages will be described here. The head, believed to be a bipyramidal hexagonal prism, has overall dimensions of 81 × 125 nm and a capacity of 3.6×10^5 nm³. It is of about 1000 S and 220 × 10^6 dalton particle weight. Some strains, e.g., T 2L, can also exist as a 15% elongated head form of 700 S which is noninfective. The contractile tail is 25 × 110 nm.

The phage head contains a linear double-stranded DNA molecule of about 54 μm length, which, assuming a 2 nm diameter, occupies about 45% of the head's capacity. The DNA is 60 S, 120 × 10^6 dalton mol. wt., and 66% (A + T), except that the cytosine is replaced by 5-hydroxymethylcytosine. Many of these bases in turn carry α-glucosyl groups (75% in T 2), a small fraction of which is diglucose (6%). The extent and nature of this glucosylation represents a point of difference between T 2, T 4, and T 6. There is also a small amount of 6-methyladenine.

The DNA of these phages is terminally redundant and circularly permuted. Thus it has no fixed terminal nucleotide sequences.

The proteins making up the T-even phage head and tail structures have in recent years been intensely studied. No significant differences in the number and molecular weights of the protein components of the T-even phages, nor in their amino acid composition were detected (Table 5). However, some of the data obtained in different laboratories concerning the molecular weights of these proteins do not agree at all well. The lysozymes produced upon infection with T 2 and T 4 have been sequenced and found very similar (Figure 6). (Cummings, 1972; Cummings *et al.*, 1970; Forrest and Cummings, 1970.)

T 3 (*Escherichia coli*). Closely related to T 7. Isometric particles of 47 nm diameter, with a short tail (10 × 15 nm), 476 S, 49 × 10^6 in particle weight. The phage contains DNA of 24 × 10^6 daltons, 11.6 μm long, 48% (G + C). (Herrlich and Schweiger, 1970.)

T 4 (*Escherichia coli*). This phage is in gross aspects identical with T 2 and T 6, and the data given there are valid also for T 4 (see Electron micrograph XVIII). The DNA is of 61 S; 119 × 10^6 mol. wt. (although more recent analysis favors lower values, e.g., 105 or 110 × 10^6, for all these large-phage DNAs); it is 52 μm long, 66% (A + T). Only the state of glucosylation differs, the hydroxymethylcytidine in T 4 being 70% α- and 30% β-glucosylated.

Protein and assembly studies have recently been performed with T 4 and have yielded the following data. The capsomeres building up the head are of 5 nm diameter and 6.2 S. The head consists of seven proteins of molecular weights above 15,000, ranging from 69,000 to 18,000, three of which have larger precursor proteins which are cleaved during maturation. The main structural proteins appear to be P23 and P24 of 46,500 and 43,500 daltons, derived from 56 and 45×10^3 dalton precursors, but a smaller internal protein of 21×10^3 daltons also arises from a precursor (23.5×10^3 daltons) during maturation. This may be the so-called internal protein (about 5% of the total) which is specific for each phage strain, and of as yet unrecognized function. The N-terminal groups of these proteins are mostly alanine and some methionine. Also, there are two distinct polypeptides amounting to about 1% and apparently also concerned with head assembly. The presence of putrescine and spermidine in the phage head in amounts equivalent to one-third of the DNA phosphate groups probably plays no specific role nor is it genetically determined.

The head appears to be attached to the tail and particularly to its thin axial tube, the so-called core or tail tube, by a protein plug at the apex of one of the pyramids, a protein of 35,000 daltons. The sheath is now believed to be formed from a single glycoprotein of 50,000–80,000 daltons lacking a free N-terminus and containing one histidine residue. There are probably 144 molecules of this protein in 24 rings. The tail tube also consists of a single protein (21,000 daltons). However, no good agreement on the nature of the tail proteins has been reached.

By far the most complicated structure is the six-pronged base plate, which seems to consist of twelve proteins ranging from 24×10^3 to 140×10^3 daltons. The tail fibers consist of two main structural proteins making up the two 70-nm-long branches of the fibers, of 155 and 120×10^3 daltons. Thus about 30 proteins make up the T-even phages, but their assembly requires at least another 15 factors such as enzymes which do not form part of the mature particle.

Among these enzymes is a lysozyme which has been studied in chemical and genetic detail. T 4 lysozyme was found to differ in only three amino acids from T 2 lysozyme, both sequences being known (Figure 6). The functional role of the lysozyme is not yet clear, nor is that of the presence of dihydrofolate reductase and pteroylhexaglutamate in the base plate, nor that of about 140 firmly bound Ca^{++} ions and ATP molecules in the contractile sheath (which consists of 144 protein molecules), the latter being released upon contraction. (Poglazov *et al.*, 1972; King and Mykolajewycz, 1973; Laemmli, 1970.)

T 5 (*Escherichia coli*). The icosahedral head of this phage is 65 nm in diameter, the noncontractile tail 10×180 nm (see Electron micrograph XIX). The particle weight is 109×10^6 daltons. The tail consists of about 45 turns of 3 nm pitch. Tail fibers and base plate are very fine and thus poorly characterized. The DNA (49 S) has a molecular weight of 75×10^6 (69% of the particle weight) and is 36 μm long. It contains no single-strand nicks. Its composition is 39% (G+C). There are at least thirteen proteins, five making up the head. The main capsid protein (65%) has a molecular weight of 32 $\times 10^3$ and minor components of 43, 30, 28, 23, 19, and 18×10^3. The major tail protein (17%) is of 51×10^3, the minor components of 140, 128, 125, 82, and 70×10^3. Only 8% of the phage's DNA is initially injected into the host, the rest only after completion of the early proteins 2–3 min later. (Zweig and Cummings, 1973.)

T 6 (*Escherichia coli*). This phage is similar to T 2 and T 4 in all known respects, except for the state of glucosylation of its hydroxymethylcytosine (3% α-glucosyl, 72% β-glucosyl-α-glucosyl, 25% unglucosylated). Its composition is 66% (A+T). It is of 1050 S and 145×10^6 particle weight (?). The proteins of T 6 were compared to those of T 2 and T 4, and no significant differences were detected (*see* T 2). For amino acid composition, see Table 5. (Cummings, 1972; Forrest and Cummings, 1970.)

T 7 (*Escherichia coli*). This phage is similar to T 3, smallest of the T phages, in dimensions and all properties; 487 S; 38×10^6 particle weight (see Electron micrograph XX). The phage is isometric with a very short tail appendage. The DNA (32 S), 12.5 μm long, has a molecular weight of 24×10^6 daltons. It contains 49% (G+C). Its terminal sequences are:

$$
\begin{array}{llll}
(5') & pAG\underline{\quad r \quad}AGA & (3') \\
(3') & TCC\underline{\quad l \quad}CTp & (5')
\end{array}
$$

(The symbols *r* and *l* are now used to designate the heavier (denser) and lighter strand, respectively.) It codes for about 30 proteins, 25 of which have been genetically and functionally identified. At least 11 are in the mature particle, ranging in molecular weight from 13 $\times 10^3$ to 150×10^3. The major head protein has a molecular weight of 38×10^3. Various enzymes have been identified in terms of peptide chains (molecular weights in parentheses) as follows: The RNA polymerase (100×10^3), ligase (40×10^3), endonuclease (13.5×10^3), lysozyme (13×10^3), DNA polymerase (81×10^3), and exonuclease (31×10^3). (Herrlich and Schweiger, 1970; Studier, 1972.)

UmV (*Ustilago maydis*). Isometric 41 nm diameter particle of five sedimentation constants (110–160 S), due to particles containing double-stranded RNA of 2.9, 2.5, 0.9, 0.4, and 0.06×10^6 daltons. (Wood, 1973.)

UX (*Bacillus subtilis*). Contains an odd base (?), 38% (G+C).

U 3 (*Escherichia coli,* strain K-12) (requiring cell wall galactose). Small isometric phage similar to but unrelated and distinctly smaller than X 174. 22 nm diameter, of 83 S (X 174: 114 S) and 4×10^6 particle weight, containing single-stranded DNA. At least four genes. (Watson and Paigen, 1971.)

VA-1 (*Vibrio cholerae* NIH 41). Hexagonal head and rigid contractile tail with thick base plate and prongs. (Weston *et al.,* 1973.)

VK (*Escherichia coli*). Member of group III of RNA phages (*see* Qβ). The coat protein has the same N-terminal Ala- and C-terminal -Tyr as that of Qβ. (Miyake *et al.,* 1971.)

VP 11 (*Streptomyces coelicolor*). Isometric head of 55 nm diameter and long contractile tail of 11×220 nm. (Dowding, 1973.)

V 6 (*Vibrio parahaemolyticus*). Filamentous phage; density in CsCl 1.32 g/ml. Contains single-stranded DNA. (Nakanishi *et al.,* 1966.)

V 12, 14 (*Vibrio parahaemolyticus*). Probably typical tailed DNA phages. (Nakanishi *et al.,* 1966.)

V 45 (*Vibrio foetidus*). Particles of 50 nm diameter with 7×240 nm noncontractile tail.

WAK (*Escherichia coli*). Typical particles with long noncontractile tail and forked tips.

WLL (*Escherichia coli*). Phage used by Schlesinger in classical virus-characterizing studies about 1934.

WT (*Rhizobium trifolii*). (Barnet, 1972.)

W 14 (*Pseudomonas acidovorans*). 85 nm particles with contractile tail of 140 nm. The buoyant density in CsCl (1.666 g/ml) and T_m (99.3°C) indicate respectively 4.5 and 73% (G+C) and suggest the presence of an unusual base. This was found to be 5-(4-

aminobutylaminomethyl)-uracil (or thyminylputrescine) partly replacing thymine (about 50%). (Kropinski *et al.*, 1973.)

W 31 (*Escherichia coli*). Similar to I, II.

Xf (*Escherichia coli*). Filamentous particles of 6 × 838 nm.

Xf (*Xanthomonas oryzae*). Filamentous particles (8.4 × 980 nm), containing single-stranded DNA (A/G/T/C = 21/33/19/28). The protein is of molecular weight 4850 (42 amino acids), lacking histidine, cysteine, methionine, and phenylalanine; rich in hydrophobic amino acids. (Marvin and Hohn, 1969.)

XP 5 (*Xanthomonas pruni*). Contains DNA of 62% (G+C).

XP 12 (*Xanthomonas oryzae*).

X 1–7 (*Salmonella typhimurium*). X 1: Particle with 66 nm diameter head and 14 × 220 nm tail with 210 nm fibers. X 7: Particle with 85 nm diameter head and 19 × 263 nm tail with 185 nm fibers.

X 174 (*Escherichia coli*). This is the prototype of the small isometric DNA phages to which belong S 13, R, and others. Phages of this group are quite similar and serologically related. These phages, in contrast to the small isometric RNA phages and the small filamentous DNA phages, do not adsorb to pili and are thus not restricted to male or other pili-carrying bacteria. In contrast to the latter, they cause lysis.

The X 174 particle has a diameter of 25 nm, a particle weight of 6.2×10^6, 114S, and a buoyant density in CsCl of 1.43 g/ml. It is icosahedral with twelve readily visible protruberances on the apices (see Electron micrograph XXI).

The DNA of X 174 (25.5%) is single-stranded and circular, with a molecular weight of 1.6×10^6. Its composition is A/G/T/C = 25/24/33/18. Its nucleotide sequence is being actively studied using in principle the same methods of specific protein binding which are being used with the RNA of phages to locate and protect specific DNA segments. Two pieces of about 50 nucleotides have been sequenced (Figure 7).

The main coat protein of X 174 and related phages, of which there are 60 molecules, is of molecular weight 48,000; it has N-terminal Ser-Asp-. The most structurally characteristic feature of these viruses are the 12 prominent capsomeres located on the apices of the icosahedron. These consist of pentamers of two proteins forming the base and one molecule of a third protein forming the apex of what might be regarded as a microtail, surely the attachment organ of these viruses. The molecular weights of these spike proteins are 19,000 (with N-terminal Met-Phe-Gln-Thr-Phe-Ile-Ser-Arg-His-, see Figure 7) and 5000, and the tip protein 36,000. Thus each of these capsomeres weighs 156,000 daltons.

The phages of the X 174 group have eight or more probably nine genes, four of which code for the proteins discussed above and the rest for functions connected with the replication and packaging of the DNA. (Robertson *et al.*, 1973; Ziff *et al.*, 1973.)

χ (*Salmonella*). Attacks the flagellae of motile *Salmonella* strains only. Icosahedral hexagonal particles of 67 nm diameter with 14×220 nm tails with 55 fine striations (pitch 4.2 nm), and a single tail fiber (2.2×210 nm). 55% (G+C). (Meynell, 1961; Schade *et al.*, 1967.)

ZG (*Escherichia coli*). Member of group IV of RNA phages; A/U = 1.05. (Miyake *et al.*, 1971.)

ZIK/1 (*Escherichia coli*). RNA phage not clearly belonging to any group. A/U = 0.83, the coat protein has a molecular weight of 12,100 and lacks histidine, methionine, and cysteine. (Robinson, 1972.)

ZJ 1 (*Escherichia coli*). Member of group I of RNA phages; A/U = 0.86 (*see* f 2).

ZJ 2 (*Escherichia coli*). Filamentous particle (6.8×830 nm) containing single-stranded DNA. Very similar and closely related to fd. The amino acid sequence of the coat protein consisting of 50 amino acid residues is discussed under fd. (Snell and Offord, 1972.)

ZL 3 (*Escherichia coli*). Member of group IV of RNA phages; A/U = 1.06. (Miyake *et al.*, 1971.)

ZR (*Escherichia coli*). Member of group I of RNA phages (*see* f 2). The coat protein contains the same N-terminal Ala- and C-terminal -Ile-Tyr as MS 2. (Miyake *et al.*, 1971.)

ZS 3 (*Escherichia coli*). Member of group IV of RNA phages; A/U = 1.06.

1 (*Bacillus subtilis*). Contains 52 S DNA of 44% (G+C). (Ito and Spizizen, 1971.)

1X1 (*Pseudomonas aeruginosa*). Contains DNA of 63% (G+C).

1ϕ7 (*Escherichia coli* and *Proteus vulgaris*). (Lisovskaya, 1972.)

2, 6, 7, 8, 9, 10 (*Pseudomonas aeruginosa*). Temperate phages (Bartell and Orr, 1969; Bartell *et al.,* 1971.)

2 (*Salmonella typhimurium*, etc.). Similar to E 1.

2 (*Bacillus subtilis*). Contains DNA with 44% (G+C).

2C (*Bacillus subtilis*). Particle weight about 100×10^6. Virus contains DNA of 40% (G+C), with 5-hydroxymethyl-U instead of T ($T_m = 77.8°C$). The buoyant density in CsCl is 1.742 g/ml, that of the two chains 1.752 and 1.762 g/ml. (Truffaut *et al.,* 1970.)

2G 3A (*Escherichia coli*).

3 (*Bacillus subtilis*). Temperate phage. Contains DNA with 36% (G+C). (Ito and Spizizen, 1971.)

3B (*Staphylococcus* B). Particles of 60×80 nm, with 300 nm tail.

3ML (*Streptococcus*). Various head sizes.

6 (*Staphylococcus* B). Particles of 40×92 nm with 300 nm tail.

6 (*Pseudomonas phaseolicola*). The phage shows a polyhedral 60 nm head covered by a lipid envelope, the lipid composition resembling that of the host. The tail is short and complex. Lipid content 25%, RNA 13%, protein 62%. Buoyant density in CsCl 1.27 g/ml. The double-stranded RNA of molecular weight 1.9, 2.8, and 4.6×10^6 averages 56% (G+C). The phage is sensitive to ether, etc. It contains RNA polymerase. (Vidaver *et al.,* 1973.)

7S (*Pseudomonas aeruginosa*). Similar and related to PP 7, icosahedral picornavirus of 25 nm diameter. (Feary *et al.,* 1964; Bradley, 1966.)

12B, 12S (*Pseudomonas syringae*). Particles with octahedral head and contractile tail with cross-striations and a few fine fibers.

14 (*Bacillus subtilis*). Contains DNA of 44% (G+C).

15 (*Bacillus subtilis*). Morphologically like 29, and sharing long nucleotide sequences. Contains DNA of 23 S, 12×10^6 mol. wt. (6.1 nm long), with 34% (G+C). At least seven proteins occur in the virion (Ito *et al.,* 1973.)

15 (*Escherichia coli*). A defective phage.

17 (*Actinomyces*). DNA of 59% (G+C).

21 (*Bacillus subtilis?*). DNA of 50% (G+C).

21 (*Escherichia coli*). Deletion mutant of λ. The DNA has the same cohesive sequences as λ. (Murray and Murray, 1973.)

25 (*Bacillus subtilis*). Contains DNA of 64 S, 43% (G+C), with 5-
hydroxymethyl-U instead of T.

29 (*Bacillus subtilis*). Unusual hexagonal head (31.5 × 41.5 nm) with
many fine projections and a 32.5 nm tail with two collars and twelve
appendages (14 nm long). The weight of the 256 S particle is 18 ×
10^6 daltons, with 56% DNA of 39% (G+C). The head is composed
of one main protein of 54 × 10^3 and two others of 48 and 28 × 10^3
mol. wt.; the neck with collar and appendages consists of three proteins (80, 40, 36 × 10^3 mol. wt.), and the tail of one protein (71 ×
10^3 mol. wt.). (Alvarez *et al.*, 1972.)

41C (*Bacillus subtilis*). Hexagonal head of 50 nm diameter with 10 ×
140 nm noncontractile tail, lacking fibers and base plate, same
(G+C) as host. (Zsigray *et al.*, 1973.)

44A (*Staphylococcus aureus* and *S. pyogenes*). Contains DNA of 27%
(G+C).

52 (*Staphylococcus* B). Particles of 50 nm diameter with 150 nm tails.

66t (*Salmonella typhimurium*). Similar to T-even phages of *E. coli*.

70 (*Staphylococcus* B). Particles of 53 × 98 nm with 300 nm tail.

77 (*Staphylococcus* B). Isometric particles of 55 nm diameter with 220
nm tail.

80 (*Staphylococcus pyogenes*). Contains DNA of 37% (G+C).

80 (*Escherichia coli*). Temperate deletion mutant related to λ; 53%
(G+C); 13.8 μm long; 30 × 10^6 mol. wt., 8% less than λ DNA. The
cohesive ends are the same as those of λ. (Bambara *et al.*, 1973;
Yamagishi and Ozeki, 1972; Deeb, 1972.)

80 (*Chlostridium perfringens*). Typical particles with short tail. (Vieu *et
al.*, 1965.)

81 (*Staphylococcus pyogenes*). Contains DNA of 35% (G+C).

82 (*Escherichia coli*). Deletion mutant, closely related to λ, with same
cohesive sequences. (Murray and Murray, 1973.)

91 (*Staphylococcus* B). Particles of 50 nm diameter with 150 nm tails.

105 (*Bacillus subtilis*). Temperate phage, incapable of generalized trans-
duction; genetically unrelated but similar to SPO 2 (slight

serological cross-reaction); inducible by mitomycin C. The head is hexagonal with 52 nm diameter, the tail 10×220 nm, equipped with hexagonal endplate, 23 nm in diameter, but no tail fibers. The DNA is of 25×10^6 mol. wt., possibly with cohesive ends. It contains 43.5% (G+C). (Rutberg *et al.*, 1972.)

149 (*Vibrio cholerae*). Particles with 75×85 nm head, 11×155 nm flexuous tail with terminal knob of 13 nm diameter and prongs. (Maiti and Chatterjee, 1971.)

186 (*Escherichia coli*). Temperate phage, related to P 2, P 4, 299, D, and N 1. Similar to but not closely related to λ, with different cohesive sequence, the left single-stranded 5′-terminal sequence of 19 nucleotides being pGGCGTGGCGGGGAAAGCAT- (the right being complementary to it). (Padmanabhan and Wu, 1972.)

299 (*Escherichia coli*). Temperate phage related to 186 and P 2, with slightly different cohesive sequence, yet able to cohere to that of 186. (Murray and Murray, 1973.)

317 (*Rhizobium leguminosarum*). Icosahedral particle of 59 nm diameter with tail carrying three fibers of 27 nm. Contains DNA of 41×10^6 mol. wt., 22 nm long, and 55% (G+C). (Ley *et al.*, 1972.)

363 (*Escherichia coli*). Temperate deletion mutant; related to λ.

424 (*Escherichia coli*). Temperate deletion mutant related to λ (not closely), with same cohesive sequence. (Murray and Murray, 1973.)

434 (*Escherichia coli*). Deletion mutant related to λ.

581 (*Staphylococcus aureus*). Particles of 55 nm with 240 nm tails.

594n (*Staphylococcus*). Particles of 55×96 nm with 300 nm non-contractile tail with knobs at the tip.

3610 (*Bacillus subtilis*). Defective phage, similar to PBSX, α or μ. Isometric 33–42 nm particle with 190–280 nm tail and 660-nm-long fibers.

8762 (*Alcaligenes faecalis*). Particles with long tails. (Maré *et al.*, 1966.)

I, II (*Escherichia coli*, female strain specific). Morphologically similar and closely related to T 7, also almost identical to H of *Pasteurella pestis*). (Williams and Meynell, 1971; Brunovskis *et al.*, 1973.)

I ϕ 7 (*Escherichia coli, Proteus vulgaris*).

VI (*Proteus mirabilis*). Virulent phage. (Wilke and Böhme, 1972.)

List of Anonymous Viruses of Protists

(In alphabetical order of their hosts)

Arthrobacter globiformis (ATCC8010). Phage AG8010 has a hexagonal head of 69 × 60 nm and a thin sheathless tail of 120 nm. Its density in CsCl is 1.534 g/ml. The DNA is 63% (G+C). (Einck *et al.*, 1973.)

Bdellovibrio bacteriovorus. Ten phage groups. Several isometric, 25 nm diameter; three with 50–75 nm heads and contractile tails of about 160 nm; also particles of 40 nm head diameter and 200 nm tail. (Schindler and Ludvik, 1972; Althauser *et al.*, 1973.)

Brucella. Many isolates. *See also* A 422, M 51, S 708, Tbilisi.

Chondrococcus columnaris (mycobacterium). Particles with contractile tails.

Corynebacteria spp. Twenty strains were described, all similar (β, ov1, ov2, ov3, cap 1, UH1, UH3, uh3, uh5, uh6, UB1, ub2, hg1, hg2, MLMa, 28, 29, 4498, IA) with 55–60 × 61–72 nm heads, 8–10 × 245–298 nm tails. (Nagington and Carne, 1971.)

Entamoeba histolytica (HB301). Polyhedral particles, assembled in perinuclear cytoplasm. Filamentous particles assembled in nucleus. (Diamond *et al.*, 1972; Mattern *et al.*, 1972).

Listeria monocytogenes. Long noncontractile tail.

Methanomonas methylovora. See MP 1–3.

Mycobacterium smegmatis. See BO 1, BO 2a, BO 2h.

Penicillium brevicompactum and *P. chrysogenum*. (*See* PcV.) Icosahedral 35–40 nm diameter particles of 147 S and 128 S; buoyant density in CsCl 1.36 g/ml. These, like AsF, PsF, etc. phages, contain double-stranded RNA (13 S) of 2.18, 1.99, and

155

1.89 × 10⁶ daltons, separately encapsidated. RNA polymerase is also detectable. (Wood and Bozarth, 1972.)

Penicillium stoloniferum. See PSVs, PSVf.

Rhizobium lupini. Six different phages have been isolated. One of these (16-2-4) has been described as consisting of a 50 nm head and a flexuous 140 nm helical tail. Their DNAs have molecular weights of 27–50 × 10⁶ and 53–62% (G+C). All were linear and some had cohesive ends. (Mayer *et al.,* 1973.)

Rhizobium trifolii (see also CT 1–6, NT 1–4, ST, WT.) Four groups of phages have been isolated. Isolates c and I have 74 nm diameter heads and 115 nm contractile tails; isolates a, e, l, and J have 82 nm diameter heads and 124 nm contractile tails; isolates j, m, and E have 110 nm diameter heads and 144 nm contractile tails; and isolates b, d, f, h, and i have 100 nm diameter heads and 330 nm noncontractile tails. The structures at the end of the tails differ within groups. (Atkins, 1973.)

Rhizobium leguminosarum. See phage 317.

Streptococcus agalactiae. Particles with 61 × 56 nm head, flexuous 7.5 × 150 nm tail. (Russell *et al.,* 1969.)

Streptococcus sanguis group H. Phages with long noncontractile particles similar to GT 234, A 25, etc. (Parsons *et al.,* 1972.)

Thiobacillus novellus. Polyhedral head of 60 nm diameter and tail (8 × 85 nm) surrounded by five filaments. Density in CsCl is 1.51 g/ml. DNA of 58% (G+C); five proteins of molecular weight 62–14 × 10³ have been detected. (Johnson *et al.,* 1973.)

Thraustochytrium (fungus). Herpes-like enveloped virus of 110 nm diameter, with a DNA-containing core, which is replicated in the nucleus. (Kazama and Schorstein, 1972.)

Ustilago maydis (fungus). *see* UmV.

TABLE 5
Amino Acid Composition of Near-Pure Phage Proteins

	Asp	Thr	Ser	Glu	Pro	Gly	Ala	Cys	Val	Met	Ile	Leu	Tyr	Phe	Lys	His	Arg	Trp	Total number
Phage λ																			
Heads	33	19	20	40	16	20	25	1	25	10	11	21	12	12	17	1	18	2	303
Tails	34	40	29	30	19	33	38	1	38	7	10	16	7	10	18	1	12	4	347
Main capsid protein of																			
Phage X 174	23	16	12	19	13	15	15	1	12	6	10	16	6	10	9	6	11	ND	>190
Phage S 13	29	14	14	18	16	16	15	1	12	ND	9	16	7	9	11	5	11	ND	>203
T-even phages																			
Tail tube	13	7.5	7	11	3.9	13	8.5	0.6	5.6	0.9	6.3	6.3	3.0	3.1	5.0	1.0	4.0	0.7	
Capsid proteins*																			
mol. wt. 43,000																			
T2	9.7	5.4	5.1	11.0	4.3	10.5	12.9	0.3	7.0	2.8	6.8	5.8	4.1	4.5	5.6	0.8	4.0	0.4	
T4	9.9	6.5	5.3	11.0	4.3	10.5	13.1	0.3	7.0	2.6	6.6	5.4	4.0	4.2	5.2	0.8	3.8	0.5*	
T6	10.0	5.5	5.4	10.7	4.3	10.4	12.8	0.3	6.7	2.8	7.0	5.8	4.0	4.4	5.1	0.8	4.0	0.3	
mol. wt. 18,000																			
Average	11.6	6.5	5.4	11.8	3.8	9.2	10.5	0.4	7.2	2.3	5.8	5.1	3.3	4.6	6.9	1.0	4.7	0.7	
mol. wt. 11,000																			
T2H	8.8	6.9	6.3	13.8	3.2	6.4	9.0	0	6.2	0.3	6.4	4.0	5.8	3.6	10.6	2.4	3.0	3.4	
T4B	8.8	7.1	6.7	14.1	3.1	6.5	9.1	0	6.1	0.2	6.2	3.8	6.0	3.6	10.8	2.4	2.9	3.3	
T6	8.6	6.8	6.4	15.1	3.2	6.3	8.9	0	6.1	0.3	6.1	3.8	5.7	3.6	10.5	2.4	2.8	3.4	

* Mole percent. Strains T2L and H and T4B and B01 respectively were averaged. The only marked differences among strains was the tryptophan in T4B01, 0.2 mole percent. ND means not determined.

```
                          10        20        30        40        50        60        70        80        90       100
pppGGGUGGGACCCCUUUCGGGGUCCUGCUCAACUUCCUGUCCGUGCUAAUGCCAUUUUUAAUGUCUUUAGCGAGACGCUACCAUGGCUAUCGCUGUAGGUAGCCGAA

         110       120       130
UUCCAUUCCUAGGAGGUUUGA·CCU·AUG·CGA·GCU·UUU·AGU·G···CU·AAG·GCC·CAA·AUC·UCA·AUC·CGG·CAU·CGG·GUA·CAA·UCC·GUA·
           (A-protein) F-Met-Arg-Ala-Phe-Ser——Ala-Lys-Ala-Gln-Ile-Ser-Ala-Met-His-Arg-Gly-Val-Gln-Ser-Val—

UGG·CCA·ACA·ACU·GGC·GCG·UAC·GUA·AAG·UCU·CCU·UUC·UCG·AUG·GUC·CAU·ACC·UUA·GAU·GCG·UUA·GCA·UUA·AUC·AGG·CAA·CGG·
Trp-Pro-Thr-Thr-Gly-Ala-Tyr-Val-Lys-Ser-Pro-Phe-Ser-Met-Val-His-Thr-Leu-Asp-Ala-Leu-Ala-Leu-Ile-Arg-Gln-Arg—

A*
        G                             C**
CUC·UCU·AGA·UAG·AGCCCUCAACCGGAGUUUGA·AGC·AUG·GCU·UCU·AAC·UUU·ACU·CAG·UUC·GUU·CUG·GUC·GAC·AAU·GGC·GGA·ACU·GGC·
Leu-Ser-Arg       (coat protein)   F-Met-Ala-Ser-Asn-Phe-Thr-Gln-Phe-Val-Leu-Val-Asp-Asn-Gly-Gly-Thr-Gly-
                                                                              10

                                             C***
GAC·GUG·ACU·GUC·GCC·CCA·AGC·AAC·UUC·GCU·GGG·GUC·GCU·GAA·UGG·AUC·AGC·UCU·AAC·UCG·CGU·UCA·CAG·GCU·UAC·AAA·
Asp-Val-Thr-Val-Ala-Pro-Ser-Asn-Phe-Ala-Gly-Val-Ala-Glu-Trp-Ile-Ser-Ser-Asn-Ser-Arg-Ser-Gln-Ala-Tyr-Lys—
            20                        30                                40

U***                              G***                 U***
GUA·ACC·UGU·AGC·GUU·CGU·CAG·AGC·UCU·GCG·CAG·AAU·CGC·AAA·UAC·ACC·AUC·AAA·GUC·GAG·GUG·CCU·AAA·GUG·GCA·ACC·CAG·
Val-Thr-Cys-Ser-Val-Arg-Gln-Ser-Ala-Gln-Asn-Arg-Lys-Tyr-Thr-Ile-Lys-Val-Pro-Val-Ala-Thr-Gln—
                50                              60                              70

                              C**       C**   U***
                                              Leu**                       90
ACU·GUU·GGU·GUA·GAG·CUU·CCU·GUA·GCC·GCA·UGG·CGU·UCG·UAC·UUA·AAU·AUG·GAA·CUA·ACC·AUU·CCA·AUU·UUC·GCU·ACG·
Thr-Val-Gly-Val-Glu-Leu-Pro-Val-Ala-Ala-Trp-Arg-Ser-Tyr-Leu-Asn-Met-Glu-Leu-Thr-Ile-Pro-Ile-Phe-Ala-Thr—
                          80

C***                                                                            120
AAU·UCC·GAC·UGC·GAC·CUU·AUU·GUU·AAG·GCA·AUG·GUU·AAG·GCA·CAA·GGU·CUC·CUA·AAA·GAU·GGA·AAC·CCG·AUU·CCC·UCA·GCA·AUC·GCA·GCA·
Asn-Ser-Asp-Cys-Glu-Leu-Ile-Val-Lys-Ala-Met-Gln-Gly-Leu-Leu-Lys-Asp-Gly-Asn-Pro-Ile-Pro-Ser-Ala-Ile-Ala-Ala—
            100                               110
```

```
           U***                    C**
AAC·UCC·GGC·AUG·UAC·UAA·UAG·AUG·CCG·GCC·AUU·CAA·ACA·UGA·GGA·UUA·CCC·AUG·UCG·AAG·ACA·ACA·AAG·UUC·AAC·UCU·
                                  129 (replicase) F-Met-Ser-Lys-Thr-Thr-Lys-
Asn-Ser-Gly-Ile-Tyr
                                                                                       -100
UUA·UGU·AUU·GAU·CUU·CCU·CGC·GAU·CUU·UCU·CUC·GAA·AUU·UAC·CAA·UCA·AUU·GCU·UCU·GUC·GCU·ACU·GG···GCUCCACCGAAAGG
     -80         -70              -60              -50              -40              -30              -20              -10
UGGGCGGGGCUUCGGCCGGACCCCUCCCUAAAGAGAGGACCCGGGAUUCUCCCGAUUUGGUAACUAGCUGCUUGGCUAGUUACCACCCA
-90
```

Unknown locations:

```
        10              20              30              40              50              60              70              80
GCUCCUACCGUAGGUAACAUGUUGCUCGGAGGCCUUACGGCCUCCGGAUGCUCCUACAUGUCAGGAACAGUUG (UUACUG)
        10              20              30              40              50
GCAUAUGAGAUGCUUACGAAGGUUCACCUUCAAGAGUUUCUUCCUAUGAG
```

In polymerase gene:

```
        10              20              30              40              50              60              70
CACAGUGACUUUACAGCAAUUGCUVACUUAAGGGACGAAUUGCUCACAAAGCAUCCGACCUAAGGUUCUGGU
        10              20              30              40              50              60  70
UAU·CGU·GAU·AUG·GUU·UAC·AUA·AAC·GAU·CGU·UUG·UCG·UCC·UGG·UCG·UCU·CUA·GGU·AUC·UUG·AAC·CCA·CUA·G···
Tyr-Arg-Asp-Met-Val-Tyr-Ile-Asn-Asp-Ala-Arg-Leu-Ala-Cys-Trp-Ser-Ser-Leu-Gly-Ile-Leu-Asn-Pro-Leu- ——
```

Fig. 3. Nucleotide sequences of the RNAs of phages of group I (MS 2, R 17, and f 2). Where the nucleotide sequences correspond to known amino acid sequences, the amino acid sequences of A-protein, coat protein, and replicase are indicated under the corresponding triplets. The sequences given are those for MS 2. Identical sequences were obtained to the extent investigated for R 17 and f 2 at the 5' and 3' ends (1 to 129, −50 to −1). Differences detected within the group (R 17, f 2, MS 2) are indicated by asterisks, as follows: Both R 17 and f 2 appear to have an A in the position marked* and concerning the subsequent sequence of about 10 nucleotides data are in part preliminary and agreement not complete for MS 2, R 17, and f 2. All other differences between MS 2 on the one hand and R 17 or f 2 on the other occur at different nucleotides as indicated by ** for f 2 and *** for R 17. A spontaneous mutation was observed in R 17 in the course of its sequence studies, i.e., the G→A which occurred 10 nucleotides upstream from the coat protein initiation codon. The only located amino acid difference between these phage coats, residue 88 being leucine in f 2, as contrasted to methionine in MS 2, R 17, and M 12, was borne out by the AUG→CUG change.

Qβ: Ala-Lys-Leu-Glu-Thr-Val-Thr-Leu-Gly-Asn-Ile-Gly-Lys-Asp-Gly-Lys-Gln-Thr-Leu-Val-Leu-Asp-Pro-Arg-Gly-

f2:   Ala-Ser-Asn-Phe " Gln-Phe-Val-Leu-Val-Asn " " Gly-Thr-Gly-Asn " Thr-Val-Ala-Pro————
fr: " Glu-Glu " " " " " Asp " Lys " "

Qβ: Val-Asn-Pro-Thr-Asn-Gly-Val-Ala-Ser-Leu-Ser-Gln-Ala-Ala-Val-Pro-Ala-Leu-Glu-Lys-Arg-Val-Thr-Val-

f2: Ser " Phe-Ala " " Gln-Trp-Ile-Ser-Ser-Asn-Ser————Arg-Ser-Gln-Ala-Tyr-Lys " " Cys
fr: " " " " " " " " "

Qβ: Ser-Val-Ser-Gln-Pro-Arg—————Asn-Arg-Lys————Asn-Thr-Lys-Val-Gln-Val-Val—————Lys-Ile-Gln-Asn-Pro-Thr-

f2: " " -Arg " Ser-Ser-Ala-Gln " " Tyr-Thr-Ile— " Glu " Pro " Val-Ala-Thr-Gln "
fr: " " " " " Asn " " " Val— " " " Val—

Qβ: Ala-Cys-Thr-Ala-Asn-Gly-Ser-Cys-Asp-Pro-Ser-Val-Thr-Arg-Gln-Ala-Tyr-Ala-Asp-Val-Thr-Phe-Ser-Phe-Thr-

f2: Val-Gly——Gly-Val-Gln-Leu————— " Val-Ala-Ala-Trp-Arg-Ser " Leu-Asn-Leu-Glu-Leu-Thr-Ile-Pro-
fr: Gln " " " " " Met " Met "

Qβ: Gln-Tyr-Ser-Thr-Asp-Glu-Glu-Arg-Ala-Phe——Val-Arg-Thr-Glu-Leu-Ala-Ala-Leu-Leu-Ala-Ser-Pro-Leu-Leu-

f2: Ile-Phe-Ala " Asn-Ser-Asp-Cys-Gln-Leu-Ile " Lys-Ala-Met-Gln-Gly-Leu " Lys-Asp-Gly-Asn-Pro-Ile-
fr: Val " " " Asx-Asp " " Ala " " " Leu " " Thr-Phe " Thr " Ile-Ala-Pro-

Qβ: Ile-Asp-Ala-Ile-Asp-Gln-Leu-Asn-Pro-Ala-Tyr

f2: Pro-Ser " " Ala-Ala-Asn-Ser-Gly-Ile "
fr: Asn-Thr " " " " " " " "

Fig. 4. The amino acid sequences of the coat proteins of RNA phages (Qβ, f 2, fr). These are arranged in a manner to show the similarities between Qβ (group III), and the two related phages of group I.

```
            10              20                    30              40          50
pppGGG(G)ACCCCCCUUUAGGGGGUCAC(AC)(AC)(CUC)AGCAGUACUUCACUGAGUAUA
                                                                          (A-

           60            70                80              90          100
AGAGGACAU·AUG·CCU·AAA·UUA·CCG·CGU·GGU·CUG·CGU·UUC·GGA·GCC·GAU·AAU·
protein)F-Met-Pro-Lys-Leu-Pro

           110           120             130            140              150
GAA·AUU·CUU·AAU·GAU·UUU·CAG·GAG·CUC·UGG·UUU·CCA·GAC·CU(UUC)U·AUC·

           160           170             180            190
GAA·UCU·UCC·GAC·ACG·CAU·CCG·UGG·UAC·ACA·CUG·AAG·GGU·CGU·GUG·UUG·

200           210           220             230            240
AAC·GCC·ACC·CUU·GAU·GAU·CGU·CUA·CCU·AAU·GUA·GGC·GGU·CGC·CAG·GUA·

250           260           270             280                  290
AGG·CGC·ACA·CUC·CAU·CGC·GUC·ACC·GUU·CCG·AUU·GC[(UU)(CU)(C)]C·AGG·

           300           310           320
CCU·UCG·UCC·GGU·AAC·AAC·CGU·UCA·GUA·UGA·UCC·CGC·AG···AUCUUGAUACUACC

UUUAGUUCGUUUAAACACGUU·CUUGAUAGUAUCUUUUUAUUAACCCAACGCGUAAAGCGUUGAAAC

UUUGGGUCAAUUUG·AUC·AUG·GCA·AAA·UUA·GAG·AC···GCU·UAG·UAA·CUA·AGG·

(coat protein)  F-Met-Ala-Lys-Leu-Glu-Thr-

                                                  -160             -140
AUG·AAA·UGC·AUG·UCU·AGG·ACA·GC···CCGUGUUCUGGCACCCUACGGGGUCUUCCAGG
(Replicase) F-Met-Ser-Lys-Thr-Ala

     -120                  -100                -80
GCACGAAGGUUGCGUCUCUACACGAGGCGUAACCUGGGGGAGGGCGCCAAUAUGGCGCCUAAUUGUG

     -60                  -40                -20
AAUAAAUUAUCACAAUUACUCUUACGAGUGAGAGGGGGAUCUGCUUUGCCCUCUCUCCUCCC(A)
```

Fig. 5. Nucleotide sequences of the RNA of Qβ phage. Where the nucleotide sequences correspond to known amino acid sequences, the corresponding amino acid sequences of A-protein, coat protein, and replicase are indicated under the corresponding triplets.

```
                5                      10                     15
H-Met-Asn-Ile-Phe-Glu-Met-Leu-Arg-Ile-Asp-Glu-Gly-Leu-Arg-Leu-Lys-
                20                     25                     30
Ile-Tyr-Lys-Asp-Thr-Glu-Gly-Tyr-Tyr-Thr-Ile-Gly-Ile-Gly-His-Leu-
                35                     40                     45
Leu-Thr-Lys-Ser-Pro-Ser-Leu-Asn-Ala-Ala-Lys-Ser-Glu-Leu-Asp-Lys-
                50                     55                     60
Ala-Ile-Gly-Arg-Asn-Cys-Asn-Gly-Val-Ile-Thr-Lys-Asp-Glu-Ala-Glu-
             65                     70                     75                     80
Lys-Leu-Phe-Asn-Gln-Asp-Val-Asp-Ala-Ala-Val-Arg-Gly-Ile-Leu-Arg-
                85                     90                     95
Asn-Ala-Lys-Leu-Lys-Pro-Val-Tyr-Asp-Ser-Leu-Asp-Ala-Val-Arg-Arg-
             100                    105                    110
Cys-Ala-Leu-Ile-Asn-Met-Val-Phe-Gln-Met-Gly-Glu-Thr-Gly-Val-Ala-
             115                    120                    125
Gly-Phe-Thr-Asn-Ser-Leu-Arg-Met-Leu-Gln-Gln-Lys-Arg-Trp-Asp-Glu-
             130                    135                    140
Ala-Ala-Val-Asn-Leu-Ala-Lys-Ser-Arg-Trp-Tyr-Asn-Gln-Thr-Pro-Asn-
          145                    150                    155                    160
Arg-Ala-Lys-Arg-Val-Ile-Thr-Thr-Phe-Arg-Thr-Gly-Thr-Trp-Asp-Ala-

Tyr-Lys-Asn-Leu-OH
```

Fig. 6. Amino acid sequence of T 2 phage lysozyme. The sequence of the corresponding T 4 protein differs only in positions 40, 41, and 151 (Ser, Val, Ala, respectively).

```
pCCCATCTTGGCTTCCTTGCTGGTCAGATTGGTCGTCTTATTACCATTT(OH)
```

(Ziff *et al.*, 1973)

```
pAGGTTTTCTGCTTAGGATTTAATC·ATG·TTT·CAG·ACT·TTT·ATT·TCT·CGC·CAC(OH)
                          F-Met-Phe-Gln-Thr-Phe-Ile-Ser-Arg-His-
```

(Robertson *et al.*, 1973)

```
          10        20        30        40        50
GGCTTTATTGCTTAATTTTGCTAATTCTTTGCCTTGCCTGTATGATTTATTGGATGGT
```

(Sanger *et al.*, 1973)

Fig. 7. Deoxynucleotide sequences of phage X 174 and f 1. The first two, pertaining to X 174, represent parts of the viral, i.e., positive, strand, including the N-terminal sequence of the 20,000 mol. wt. component of the spikes of the X 174 phage. The third represents an intercistronic region of f 1 and is also given as the positive strand.

References (Section C)

Adler, R., and Pootjes, C., 1972, *J. Virol* **10**, 816.

Adolph, K. W., and Haselkorn, R., 1971, *Virology* **46**, 200.

Adolph, K. W., and Haselkorn, R., 1973, *Virology* **53**, 230.

Althauser, M., Samsonoff, W. A., Anderson, C., and Conti, S. F., 1973, *J. Virol.* **10**, 516.

Alvarez, G., Salas, E., Pérez, N., and Celis, J. E., 1972, *J. Gen. Virol.* **14**, 243.

Atkins, G. J., 1973, *J. Virol.* **12**, 149.

Bambara, R., Padmanabhan, R., and Wu, R., 1973, *J. Molec. Biol.* **75**, 741.

Banks, G. T., Buck, K. W., Chain, E. B., Darbyshire, J. E., Himmelweit, F., and Ratti, G., 1970, *Nature* **227**, 505.

Barnet, Y. M., 1972, *J. Gen. Virol.* **15**, 1.

Barrett, K., Calendar, R., Gibbs, W., Goldstein, R. N., Lindqvist, B., and Six, E., 1973, *Prog. Med. Virol.* **15**, 309.

Bartell, P. F., and Orr, T. E., 1969, *J. Virol.* **3**, 290.

Bartell, P. F., Orr, T. E., Reese, J. F., and Imaeda, T., 1971, *J. Virol.* **8**, 311.

Bendis, I., and Shapiro, L., 1970, *J. Virol.* **6**, 847.

Bertani, L. E., and Bertani, G., 1971, *Adv. Genet.* **16**, 199.

Boling, M E., Allison, D. P., and Setlow, J. K., 1973, *J. Virol.* **11**, 585.

Bradley, D. E., 1966, *J. Gen. Microbiol.* **45**, 83.

Bradley, D. E., 1967, *Bacteriol. Rev.* **31**, 230.

Bradley, D. E., 1972, *Biochem. Biophys. Res. Comm.* **47**, 142.

Bradley, D. E. 1973, *Virology* **51**, 489.

Brown, D. T., Brown, N. C., and Burlingham, B. T., 1972, *J. Virol.* **9**, 664.

Brownell, G. H., and Adams, J. N., 1967, *J. Gen. Microbiol.* **47**, 247.

Bruce, J., Gourlay, R. N., Hull, R., and Garwes, D. J., 1972, *J. Gen. Virol.* **16**, 215.

Brunovskis, I., Hyman, R. W., and Summers, W. C., 1973, *J. Virol.* **11**, 306.

Buchwald, M., Steed-Glaister, P., and Siminovitch, L., 1970, *Virology* **42**, 375.

Buck, K. W., and Kempson-Jones, G. F., 1973, *J. Gen. Virol.* **18**, 223.

Burchard, R. P., and Voelz, H., 1972, *Virology* **48**, 555.

Coetzee, J. N., Smit, J. A., and Prozesky, O. W., 1966, *J. Gen. Microbiol.* **44**, 167.

Colón, A. E., Cole, R. M., and Leonard, C. G., 1971, *J. Virol.* **8**, 103.

Contreras, R., Ysebaert, M., Min Jou, W., and Fiers, W., 1973, *Nature New Biol.* **241**, 99.

Cordes, S., Epstein, H. T., and Marmur, J., 1961, *Nature* **191**, 1097.

Coyette, J., and Calberg-Bacq, C.-M., 1967, *J. Gen. Virol.* **1**, 13.

Cummings, D. J., 1972, *J. Virol.* **9**, 547.

Cummings, D. J., Kusy, A. R., Chapman, V. A., DeLong, S. S., and Stone, K. R., 1970, *J. Virol.* **6,** 534.

Deeb, S. S., 1972, *J. Virol.* **9,** 174.

de Ley, J., Gillis, M., Pootjes, C. F., Kersters, K., Tytgat, R., and Van Braekel, M., 1972, *J. Gen. Virol.* **16,** 199.

Diamond, L. S., Mattern, C. F. T., and Bartgis, I. L., 1972, *J. Virol.* **9,** 326.

Domingo, E., Gordon, C. N., and Warner, R. C., 1972, *Virology* **49,** 439.

Donelli, G., Guglielmi, F., and Paoletti, L., 1972, *J. Molec. Biol.* **71,** 113.

Dowding, J. E., 1973, *J. Gen. Microbiol.* **76,** 163.

Dunleavy, J. M., and Urs, N. V. R., 1973, *J. Virol.* **12,** 188.

Egbert, L. N., 1972, *Biochim. Biophys. Acta* **281,** 310.

Einck, K. H., Pattee, P. A., Holt, J. G., Hagedorn, C., Miller, J. A., and Berryhill, D. L., 1973, *J. Virol.* **12,** 1031.

Eiserling, F. A., and Romig, W. R., 1962, *J. Ultrastruct. Res.* **6,** 540.

Feary, T. W., Fisher, E., and Fisher, T. N., 1964, *J. Bact.* **87,** 196.

Fedoroff, N. V., and Zinder, N. D., 1973, *Nature New Biol.* **241,** 105.

Forrest, G. L., and Cummings, D. J., 1970, *J. Virol.* **8,** 41.

Godson, G. N., 1973, *J. Molec. Biol.* **77,** 467.

Gourlay, R. N., Bruce, J., and Garwes, D. J., 1971, *Nature New Biol.* **229,** 118.

Gourlay, R. N., Garwes, D. J., Bruce, J., and Wyld, S. G., 1973, *J. Gen. Virol.* **18,** 127.

Gratia, J. P., 1973, *Molec. Gen. Genet.* **124,** 157.

Haas, M., and Yoshikawa, H., 1969, *J. Virol.* **3,** 233.

Harrison, S. C., Caspar, D. L. D., Camerini-Otero, R. D., and Franklin, R. M., 1971, *Nature New Biol.* **229,** 197.

Henry, T. J., and Brinton, C. C. Jr., 1971, *Virology* **46,** 754.

Herrlich, P., and Schweiger, M., 1970, *J. Virol.* **6,** 750.

Humbert, R. D., and Fields, M. L., 1972, *J. Virol.* **9,** 397.

Ikeda, H., and Tomizawa, J. -I., 1965, *J. Molec. Biol.* **14,** 85.

Ito, J., and Spizizen, J., 1971, *J. Virol.* **7,** 515.

Ito, J., Meinke, W., Hathaway, G., and Spizizen, J., 1973, *Virology* **56,** 110.

Jesaitis, M. A., and Hutton, J. J., 1963, *J. Exp. Med.* **117,** 285.

Johnson, K., Chow, C. T., Lyric, R. M., and van Caeseele, L., 1973, *J. Virol.* **12,** 1160.

Kay, D., and Wakefield, A. E., 1972, *J. Gen. Virol.* **14,** 271.

Kazama, F. Y., and Schorstein, K. L., 1972, *Science* **177,** 696.

Khatoon, H., Iyer, R. V., and Iyer, V. N., 1972, *Virology* **48,** 145.

King, J., and Mykolajewycz, N., 1973, *J. Molec. Biol.* **75,** 339.

King, J., Lenk, E. V., and Bottstein, D., 1973, *J. Molec. Biol.* **80,** 697.

Kisseleva, N. P., and Tikhonenko, T. I., 1972, *Biokhimiya* **37,** 562.

Kizer, P. E., and Saunders, G. F., 1972, *Biochemistry* **11,** 1562.

Knovicka, J., Pope, L., and Wyss, O., 1972, *J. Virol.* **10,** 150.

Königsberg, W., Maita, T., Katze, J., and Weber, K., 1970, *Nature* **227,** 271.

Kozloff, L. M., Raj, C. V. S., Rao, R. N., Chapman, V. A., and Delong S., 1972, *J. Virol.* **9,** 390.

Kraiss, J. P., Gelbart, S. M., and Juhasz, S. E., 1973, *J. Gen. Virol.* **20,** 75.

Kropinski, A. M. B., Bose, R. J., and Warren, R. A. J., 1973, *Biochemistry* **12,** 151.

Laemmli, V. K., 1970, *Nature* **227,** 680.

LaMontagne, J. R., and McDonald, W. C., 1972, *J. Virol.* **9,** 646.

Lengyel, J. A., Goldstein, R. N., Marsh, M., Sunshine, M. G., and Calendar, R., 1973, *Virology* **53**, 1.

Leonard, K. R., Kleinschmidt, A. K., Agabian-Keshishian, N., Shapiro, L., and Maizel, J. V. Jr., 1972, *J. Molec. Biol.* **71**, 201.

Levner, M. H., and Cozzarelli, N. R., 1972, *Virology* **48**, 402.

Ley, A. N., Warner, H. R., and Kahn, P. L., 1972, *Canad. J. Microbiol.* **18**, 375.

Lisovskaya, K. V., 1972, *Zh. Mikrobiol. Epidemiol. Immunobiol.* **49**, 80.

Liss, A., and Maniloff, J., 1971, *Science* **173**, 725.

Lomovskaya, N. D., Mkrtumian, N. M., Gostimskaya, N. L., and Danilenko, V. N., 1972, *J. Virol.* **9**, 258.

Losick, R., and Robbins, P. W., 1967, *J. Molec. Biol.* **30**, 445.

Lovett, P. S., 1972, *Virology* **47**, 743.

Mackenzie, J. J., and Haselkorn, R., 1972, *Virology* **49**, 497.

Maiti, M., and Chatterjee, S. N., 1971, *J. Gen. Virol.* **13**, 327.

Male, C. J., and Christensen, J. R., 1970, *J. Virol.* **6**, 727.

Manasse, R. J., Staples, R. C., Granados, R. R., and Barnes, E. G., 1972, *Virology* **47**, 375.

Maré, I. J., de Klerk, H. C., and Prozesky, O. W., 1966, *J. Gen. Microbiol.* **44**, 23.

Marmur, J., Brandon, C., Neubort, S., Ehrlich, M., Mandel, M., and Konvicka, J., 1972, *Nature New Biol.* **239**, 68.

Martuscelli, J., Taylor, A. L., Cummings, D. J., Chapman, V. A., Delong, S. S., and Cañedo, L., 1971, *J. Virol.* **8**, 551.

Marvin, D. A., and Hoffmann-Berling, H., 1963, *Nature* **197**, 517.

Marvin, D. A., and Hohn, B., 1969, *Bacterial Rev.* **33**, 172.

Mathews, M. M., Miller, P. A., and Pappenheimer, A. M. Jr., 1966, *Virology* **29**, 402.

Mattern, C. F. T., Diamond, L. S., and Daniel, W. A., 1972, *J. Virol.* **9**, 342.

Mayer, F., Lotz, W., and Lang, D., 1973, *J. Virol.* **11**, 946.

Meynell, E. W., 1961, *J. Gen. Microbiol.* **25**, 253.

Meynell, G. G., and Lawn, A. M., 1968, *Nature* **217**, 1184.

Milne, R. G., Thompson, G. W., and Taylor-Robinson, D., 1972, *Arch. ges. Virusforsch.* **37**, 378.

Minamishima, Y., Takeya, K., Ohnishi, Y., and Amako, K., 1968, *J. Virol.* **2**, 208.

Mise, K., 1971, *J. Virol.* **7**, 168.

Miyake, T., Haruna, I., Itoh, Y. H., Yamane, K., and Watanabe, I., 1971, *Proc. Nat. Acad. Sci.* **68**, 2022.

Morris, J. A., Corbel, M. J., and Phillip, J. I. H., 1973, *J. Gen. Virol.* **20**, 63.

Murialdo, H., and Siminovitch, L., 1972, *Virology* **48**, 785.

Murray, K., and Murray, N. E., 1973, *Nature New Biol.* **243**, 134.

Nagington, J., and Carne, H. R., 1971, *J. Gen. Virol.* **13**, 167.

Nakanishi, H., Iida, Y., Maeshima, T., Teramoto, T., Hosaka, Y., and Oraki, M., 1966, *Biken J.* **9**, 149.

Nikolskaya, I. I., Tikhonenko, T. I., Guschin, B. V., and Korzhenko, V. K., 1972, *Vopr. Virusol.* **17**, 294.

Nikolskaya, I. I., Trushinskaya, G. N., and Tikhonenko, T. I., 1972, *Biokhimiya* **37**, 101.

Nishihara, T., and Watanabe, I., 1967, *Virus,* **17**, 118.

Notani, N. K., Seflon, J. K., and Allison, D. P., 1973, *J. Molec. Biol.* **76**, 581.

Novick, R., 1967, *Virology* **33**, 155.

Nutter, R. L., Bullas, L. R., and Schultz, R. L., 1970, *J. Virol.* **5**, 754.

Okamoto, K., Mudd, J. A., Huang, W. H., Subbaiah, T. V., and Marmur, J., 1968, *J. Molec. Biol.* **34,** 413.

Oki, T., Nishida, H., and Ozaki, A. 1972, *J. Virol.* **9,** 544.

Padmanabhan, R., and Wu, R., 1972, *J. Molec. Biol.* **65,** 447.

Panter, R. A., and Symons, R. A., 1966, *Austral. J. Biol. Sci.* **19,** 565.

Parsons, C. L., Colon, A. E., Leonard, C. G., and Cole, R. M., 1972, *J. Virol.* **9,** 876.

Pemberton, J. M., 1973, *Virology* **55,** 558.

Petrovskii, I. V., Naroditskii, B. S., and Tikhonenko, T. I., 1970, *Biokhimia* **35,** 911.

Poglazov, B. F., Rodikova, L. P., and Sultanova, R. A., 1972, *J. Virol.* **10,** 810.

Poljak, R. J., and Suruda, A. J., 1969, *Virology* **39,** 145.

Pons, F. W., 1966, *Biochem. Z.* **346,** 26.

Price, A. R., and Cook, S. J., 1972, *J. Virol.* **9,** 602.

Rabussay, D., Zillig, W., and Herrlich, P., 1970, *Virology* **41,** 91.

Ratti, G., and Buck, K. W., 1972, *J. Gen. Virol.* **14,** 165.

Riva, S. C., 1969, *Biochem. Biophys. Res. Comm.* **34,** 824.

Robertson, H. D., Barrell, B. G., Weith, H. L., and Donelson, J. E., 1973, *Nature New Biol.* **241,** 38.

Robinson, J. W., 1972, *Biochem. J.* **128,** 481.

Roslycky, E. B., Allan, O. N., and McCoy, E., 1963, *Canad. J. Microbiol.* **9,** 199.

Rosner, J. L., 1972, *Virology* **48,** 679.

Russell, H., Norcross, N. L., and Kahn, D. E., 1969, *J. Gen. Virol.* **5,** 315.

Rutberg, L., Armentrout, R. W., and Jonasson, J., 1972, *J. Virol.* **9,** 732.

Safferman, R. S., Diener, T. O., Desjardins, P. R., and Morris, M. E., 1972, *Virology* **47,** 105.

Sanger, F., Donelson, J. E., Coulson, A. R., Kössel, H., and Fischer, D., 1973, *Proc. Nat. Acad. Sci.* **70,** 1209.

Schade, S. Z., Adler, J., and Ris, H., 1967, *J. Virol.* **1,** 599.

Schindler, J., and Ludvik, J., 1972, *Acta Virol.* **16,** 501.

Scott, J. R., and Shuster, R. C., 1973, *Virology* **53,** 484.

Sherman, L. A., and Haselkorn, R., 1970, *J. Virol.* **6,** 820.

Shinozawa, T., 1973, *Virology* **54,** 427.

Sinha, R. K., Misra, D. N., and Das Gupta, N. N., 1973, *Virology* **51,** 493.

Snell, D. T., and Offord, R. E., 1972, *Biochem. J.* **127,** 167.

Souza, K. A., Ginoza, H. S., and Haight, R. D., 1972, *J. Virol.* **9,** 851.

Stirm, S., and Freund-Mölbert, E., 1971, *J. Virol.* **8,** 330.

Strniste, G. F., and Taylor, W. D., 1972, *J. Virol.* **10,** 1031.

Studier, F. H., 1972, *Science* **176,** 367.

Taketo, A., and Kuno, S., 1969, *J. Biochem. (Japan)* **65,** 361.

Takeya, K., and Amako, K., 1966, *Virology* **28,** 163.

Tikhonenko, T. I., Velikodvorskaya, G. A., Bobkova, A. F., and Bartashevich, Y. E., 1973, *Nature New Biol.* in press.

Truffaut, N., Revet, B., and Soule, M.-O., 1970, *Europ. J. Biochem.* **15,** 391.

van Frank, R. M., Ellis, L. F., and Kleinschmidt, W. J., 1971, *J. Gen. Virol.* **12,** 33.

Velikodvorskaya, G. A., Bobkova, A. F., Petrovskii, G. V., and Tikhonenko, T. I., 1972, *Vopr. Virusol.* **17,** 332.

Vidaver, A. K., Koski, R. K., and Van Etten, J. L., 1973, *J. Virol.* **11,** 799.

Vieu, J. F., Guelin, A., and Daugnet, C., 1965, *Ann. Inst. Pasteur* **109,** 157.

Watanabe, H., and August, J. T., 1968, *J. Molec. Biol.* **33,** 1.

Watson, G., and Paigen, K., 1971, *J. Virol.* **8,** 669.

Weigel, P. H., England, P. T., Murray, K., and Old, R. W., 1973, *Proc. Nat. Acad. Sci.* **70**, 1151.

Weissmann, C., Billeter, M. A., Goodman, H. M., Hindley, J., and Weber, H., 1973, *Ann. Rev. Biochem.* **42**, 3031.

Weston, L., Drexler, H., and Richardson, S. H., 1973, *J. Gen. Virol.* **21**, 155.

Wilke, W., and Böhme, H., 1972, *Mutation Res.* **16**, 133.

Williams, L., and Meynell, G. G., 1971, *Molec. Gen. Genet.* **113**, 222.

Wiseman, R. L., Dunker, A. K., and Marvin, D. A., 1972, *Virology* **48**, 230.

Wittmann-Liebold, B., 1966, *Z. Naturforsch.* **21b**, 1249.

Wood, H. A., 1973, *J. Gen. Virol.* **20** (suppl.), 61.

Wood, H. A., and Bozarth, R. F., 1972, *Virology* **47**, 604.

Yamagishi, H., and Ozeki, H., 1972, *Virology* **48**, 316.

Yelton, D. B., and Thorne, C. B., 1971, *J. Virol.* **8**, 242.

Ziff, E. B., Sedat, J. W., and Galibet, F., 1973, *Nature New Biol.* **241**, 34.

Zsigray, R. M., Miss, A. L., and Landman, O. E., 1973, *J. Virol.* **11**, 69.

Zweig, M., and Cummings, D. J., 1973, *Virology* **51**, 443.

Electron
Micrographs

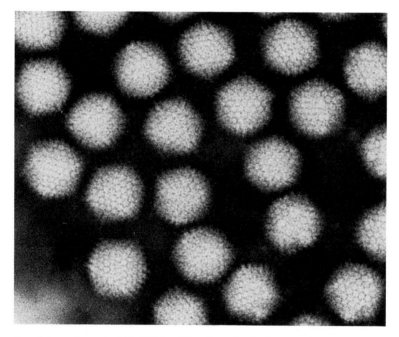

I. Adenovirus ($\times$180,000). The icosahedral arrangement of the capsomeres (hexons and pentons) is clearly visible in some particles, as are a few of the fibers (e.g., bottom left).

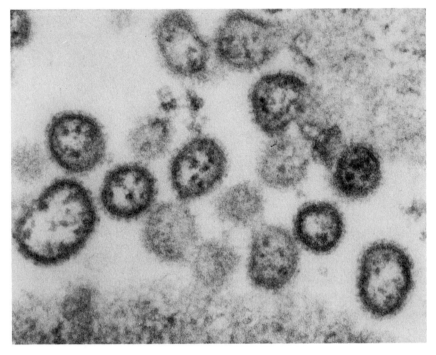

II. Arenavirus (×145,000). Lassa virus particles. The characteristic "sand grains," probably host ribosomes, are visible, as well as the membrane with peplomers.

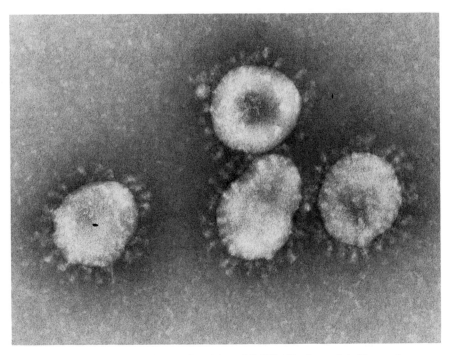

III. Coronavirus (×225,000). Particles of OC43. The long club-like peplomers represent the characteristic feature of this group of viruses.

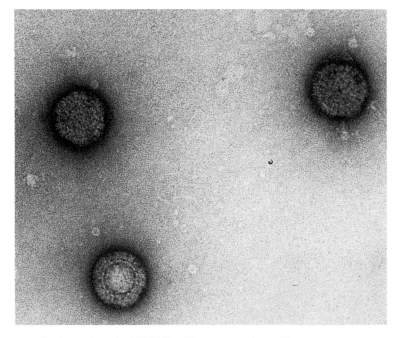

IV. Diplornavirus ($\times$150,000).   Human reovirus. The capsomeres are more clearly visible in the top particles, the double shell in the particle at the bottom.

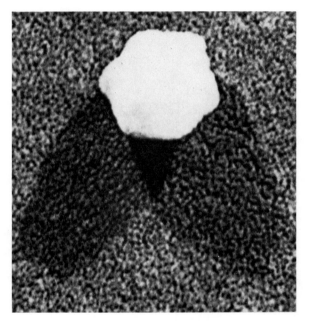

V. Iridescent virus (×220,000).   Tipula iridescent virus.
The icosahedral shape of this large virus is clearly
demonstrated by the shadows thrown in two directions.

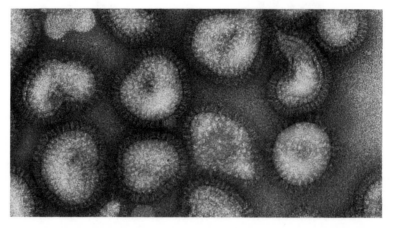

VI.   Myxovirus ($\times$170,000).   Influenza virus particles. Some pleomorphism and the dense uniform carpet of peplomers (spikes) is evident.

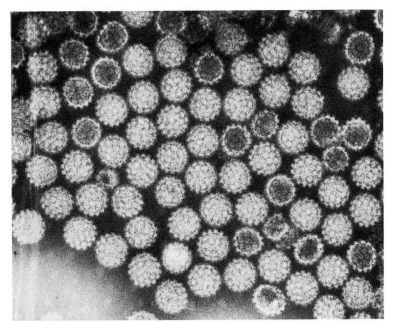

VII. Papilloma virus (×150,000).   The capsomeres of rabbit papilloma viruses are clearly evident. There are also a few empty particles.

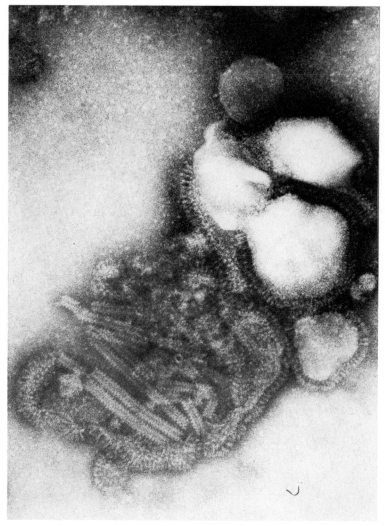

VIII. Paramyxovirus (×172,000). Sendai virus. Intact particles with peplomers as well as the helical nucleocapsids of ruptured particles are evident.

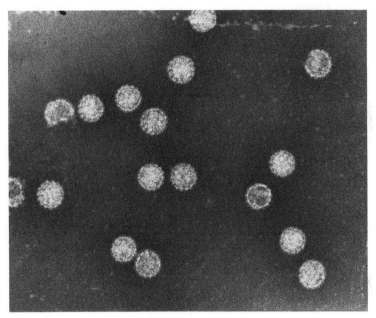

IX. Polyoma virus (×150,000). SV-40 particles, some showing the capsomeres clearly, one apparently empty.

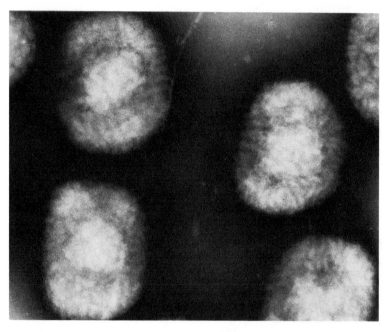

X. Poxvirus (×120,000).   Vaccinia virus particles showing some of the
typical interior features (nucleoid and lateral bodies).

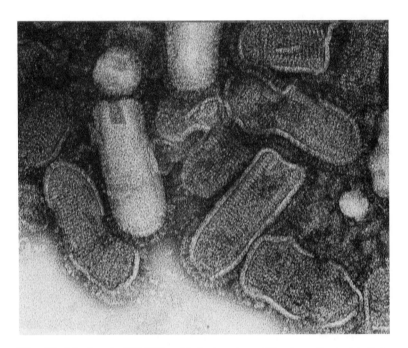

XI. Rhabdovirus ($\times$ 200,000).   Vesicular stomatitis virus. Typical bullet-shaped particles with envelope, peplomers, evident internal helical nucleocapsid. Some pleomorphism is evident.

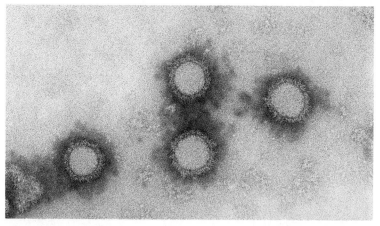

XII.   Togavirus ($\times$140,000).   Sindbis virus. The toga or cloak is clearly set off, probably because it represents the glycoproteins resting on a very lipid-rich membrane covering the nucleocapsid.

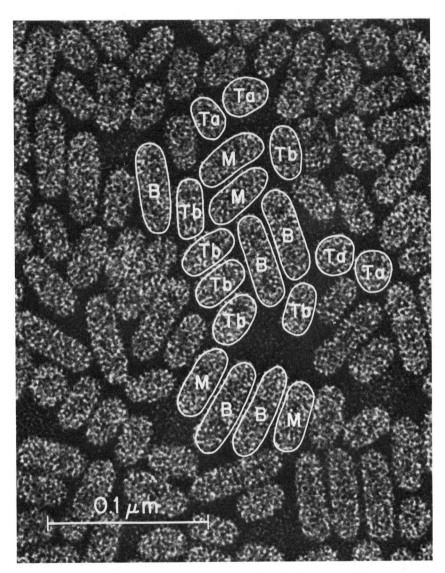

XIII. Alfalfa mosaic virus. B, M, Ta, and Tb signify bottom, middle, and top components.

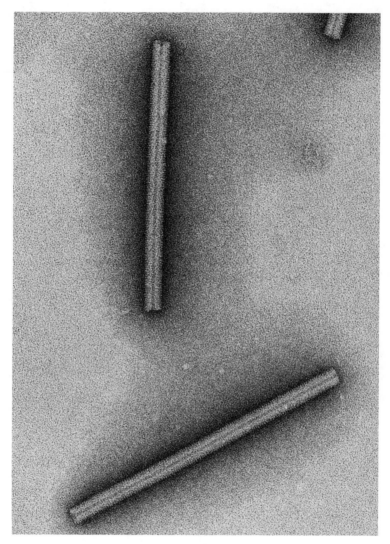

XIV. Tobacco mosaic virus ($\times$260,000).   The helical arrangement of the nucleocapsid and the axial canal is evident. Also with some imagination a neater and a less neat end of each rod can be discerned.

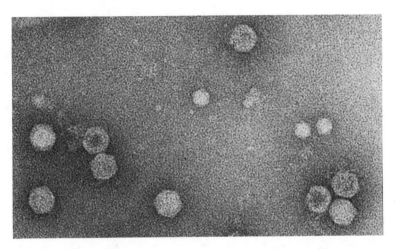

XV. Tobacco necrosis virus and satellite tobacco necrosis (the three small particles) (×250,000). The icosahedral shape is evident in both types of particles. Some of the tobacco necrosis particles appear to be empty.

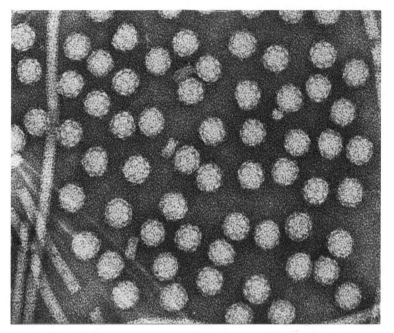

XVI.   Turnip yellows mosaic virus ($\times 250,000$).   The (32) capsomeres are clearly evident. On the left are parts of a few filamentous particles of potato virus X, showing characteristic helical capsid formation.

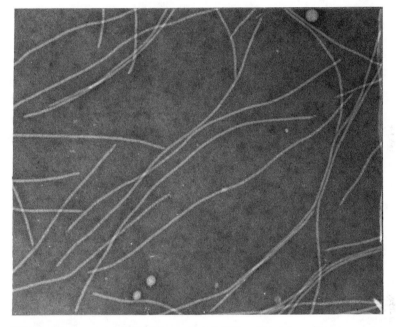

XVII. Filamentous bacteriophage ($\times$100,000).   Particles of fd phage. At this magnification, which allows entire particles to be shown, no detail is apparent, except possibly a difference in the appearance of the two ends of these particles.

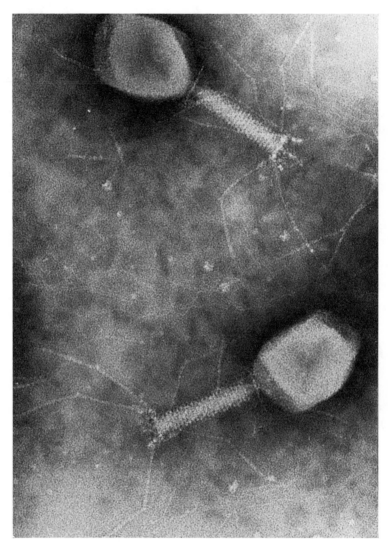

XVIII.   T-even bacteriophage (T 4) (×250,000).   The helical tail sheath, the base plate with pins, and the tail fibers are particularly evident.

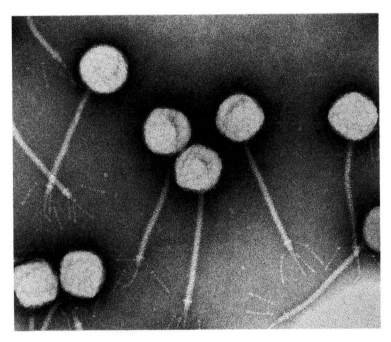

XIX. T 5 bacteriophage ($\times$150,000). Typical phage with long non-contractile tails. Helical tail structure with typical base plate with prong and fibers.

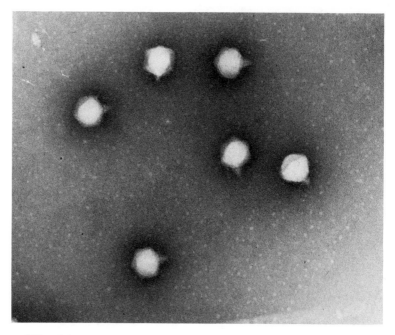

XX. T 7 bacteriophage ($\times$130,000).   Typical phage with short non-contractile tail. Icosahedral symmetry is the only noticeable feature.

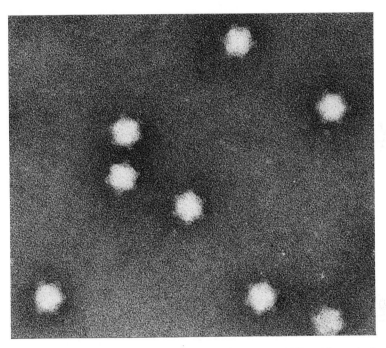

XXI. Isometric DNA bacteriophage (X 174) ($\times$240,000). The apical protuberances, now known to consist of eleven protein molecule of three types, can be seen.